Independent Medical Lab Technician Study Guide 2027-2028:

400 Practice Questions with Step-by-Step Explanations, Lab Procedures and Exam Prep Strategies for MLT Exam

Yolanda Mensah

Author Introduction

Precision in the laboratory is more than a technical skill—it is a responsibility that directly influences patient care, clinical decisions, and public health outcomes. The Medical Laboratory Technician (MLT) examination represents a critical milestone for aspiring professionals who seek to uphold the highest standards of diagnostic accuracy and scientific integrity. This study guide has been developed with that responsibility in mind.

The author of this guide is an experienced laboratory professional and educator who has worked extensively in clinical laboratory environments, supporting both routine diagnostic testing and complex analytical procedures. With a deep understanding of hematology, microbiology, clinical chemistry, immunology, and laboratory operations, the author brings practical insight into the competencies required for success on the Medical Laboratory Technician exam. This expertise is strengthened through close collaboration with a dedicated team of subject matter specialists, laboratory supervisors, and allied health educators who collectively ensure that every chapter reflects current standards, best practices, and exam-aligned expectations.

Recognizing that candidates often balance rigorous coursework, clinical rotations, and professional responsibilities, this guide has been carefully structured to promote clarity, efficiency, and mastery. Complex topics are broken down into manageable explanations without sacrificing scientific depth. Emphasis is placed not only on memorization of key concepts, but on understanding laboratory principles, quality control procedures, instrumentation, safety protocols, and result interpretation—skills that are essential both for examination success and for real-world laboratory performance.

The author and contributing team share a unified commitment to student achievement. Each section has been designed to reinforce foundational knowledge while strengthening critical thinking and problem-solving abilities. Practice-focused explanations anticipate common areas of difficulty and address them directly, enabling readers to build confidence alongside competence. Special attention has been given to aligning content with current competency standards and the analytical reasoning required in modern laboratory practice.

Above all, this study guide reflects a belief that well-prepared Medical Laboratory Technicians play an indispensable role in healthcare delivery. By combining professional experience, collaborative expertise, and a dedication to educational excellence, the author aims to provide candidates with a reliable, comprehensive resource that supports both examination readiness and long-term professional growth in the clinical laboratory field.

Table of Content

Chapter 1 - Blood Banking

Principles of Immunohematology

Blood banking rests upon the science of immunohematology—the study of antigen-antibody reactions involving red blood cells. This discipline provides the foundation for safe transfusion practice, emphasizing the recognition of antigenic structures on erythrocyte membranes and the detection of antibodies within serum or plasma. Each person's blood group antigens, inherited through Mendelian genetics, determine compatibility and guide donor selection. The central principle is that agglutination or hemolysis results when incompatible red cells encounter antibodies directed against their surface antigens. Laboratory testing in immunohematology focuses on reproducing these reactions in vitro under controlled conditions to predict in vivo responses. Understanding the strength, specificity, and clinical significance of antibodies allows technologists to differentiate harmless cold-reacting agglutinins from those capable of causing hemolytic transfusion reactions or hemolytic disease of the newborn. In essence, immunohematology translates immunologic theory into the protection of patient safety through precise laboratory technique and interpretive skill.

ABO Blood Group System

The ABO system forms the cornerstone of transfusion compatibility testing. It classifies human blood based on the presence or absence of A and B antigens on red cells and the corresponding naturally occurring antibodies in plasma. Type A individuals possess the A antigen and anti-B antibody, type B possess the B antigen and anti-A antibody, type AB have both antigens but lack antibodies, and type O lack both antigens while producing both antibodies. These reactions are so predictable that the ABO grouping is considered the single most critical determination in pretransfusion testing. Discrepancies between forward typing (antigen detection) and reverse typing (antibody confirmation) must be resolved before any blood issue, as even minor errors can lead to catastrophic hemolytic reactions. The discovery of the ABO system revolutionized transfusion medicine by transforming what was once a dangerous procedure into a routine life-saving therapy.

Rh Blood Group System

Second only to ABO in clinical significance, the Rh system primarily concerns the D antigen, a potent immunogen found on red cell membranes. Individuals expressing this antigen are designated Rh positive, whereas those lacking it are Rh negative. The Rh factor gained historical importance when sensitized Rh-negative mothers produced antibodies against Rh-positive fetal cells, resulting in hemolytic disease of the newborn. Laboratory testing involves both direct antigen typing and indirect antibody screening to detect potential sensitization. Unlike ABO antibodies, which occur naturally, Rh antibodies develop only after exposure through transfusion or pregnancy. Careful matching of Rh type between donor and recipient is essential to prevent alloimmunization and transfusion reactions. Advances in molecular testing now allow genotyping of Rh variants, improving the accuracy of compatibility testing in complex serologic cases.

Antibody Screening and Identification

The detection of unexpected antibodies forms the backbone of safe transfusion practice. Antibody screening tests determine whether a patient's plasma contains clinically significant antibodies directed against common red cell antigens other than ABO and Rh. If the screen is positive, antibody identification follows, involving testing against a panel of reagent cells with known antigen profiles. Technologists interpret reaction patterns to deduce antibody specificity, such as anti-Kell, anti-Duffy, or anti-Kidd. The process demands patience, reasoning, and correlation with transfusion and pregnancy history. Temperature, phase of testing, and reaction strength all help differentiate between cold and warm antibodies. Only through meticulous antibody identification can compatible units be selected, ensuring that transfused cells survive and function as intended.

Crossmatching Procedures

Crossmatching represents the final pretransfusion check of donor-recipient compatibility. It involves mixing the patient's serum with donor red cells to detect any reaction that might not have appeared during screening. The major crossmatch assesses recipient serum against donor cells, whereas the minor crossmatch, once common, is now largely redundant due to universal donor screening. In modern practice, an electronic crossmatch may substitute for serologic testing when antibody screens are negative and patient history is uncomplicated. However, the principle remains unchanged: no unit should be transfused unless compatibility is assured. The crossmatch confirms both laboratory accuracy and immunologic safety, serving as the last safeguard between laboratory procedure and patient bedside.

Blood Component Preparation and Storage

Blood collected from donors is separated into components—red blood cells, plasma, platelets, and cryoprecipitate—each tailored to specific clinical needs. This process maximizes the utility of each donation while reducing the risk of volume overload and immune reactions. Preparation requires sterile technique, controlled centrifugation, and precise labeling to preserve product identity. Storage conditions are strictly regulated: red cells are maintained at refrigerated temperatures, platelets at controlled room temperature with agitation, and plasma products are frozen to maintain clotting factor stability. Expiration dating, additive solutions, and leukoreduction technologies ensure that each unit remains viable and safe. Adherence to these standards exemplifies the precision and accountability inherent in blood banking practice.

Transfusion Reactions and Investigation

Despite rigorous testing, transfusion reactions can occur and demand immediate investigation. Reactions may be acute or delayed, immune or nonimmune, hemolytic or nonhemolytic. The hallmark of effective investigation is prompt recognition of clinical signs such as fever, chills, hemoglobinuria, or hypotension. Laboratory evaluation includes clerical checks, repeat ABO and Rh testing, direct antiglobulin testing, and inspection of plasma for hemolysis. Identifying the cause prevents recurrence and protects both current and future recipients. The technologist's ability to correlate serologic evidence with patient symptoms demonstrates the critical intersection between laboratory science and clinical medicine. Each reaction is a reminder that vigilance remains the defining quality of transfusion safety.

Quality Control and Regulatory Compliance

Blood bank operations function under strict regulatory oversight to ensure accuracy, traceability, and patient protection. Quality control measures verify reagent reactivity, instrument calibration, temperature monitoring, and record integrity. Every step, from donor collection to product issuance, must meet standards established by accrediting agencies and national regulations. Documentation is both a scientific and legal safeguard. Technologists perform daily checks, review reaction trends, and participate in proficiency testing to maintain continual readiness. Regulatory compliance transcends routine—it represents a professional ethic of reliability and accountability that defines the laboratory's contribution to patient care.

Automation and Molecular Advances

Modern blood banking increasingly relies on automation and molecular diagnostics to enhance accuracy and efficiency. Automated analyzers perform blood grouping, antibody screening, and crossmatching with minimal manual intervention, reducing error potential and standardizing results. Molecular genotyping now complements serologic testing by identifying variant alleles and silent antigens undetectable by conventional methods. These technologies facilitate complex transfusion support, particularly in patients with multiple antibodies or chronic transfusion needs. Automation does not replace professional judgment but augments it, freeing technologists to focus on interpretation, quality assurance, and problem-solving. The integration of molecular and automated systems marks a new era in immunohematology, where precision and speed coexist in the service of patient safety.

Ethical and Professional Responsibilities

The practice of blood banking carries profound ethical responsibility. Each unit of blood represents a human donation intended to sustain another life. Laboratory professionals must honor this trust by upholding standards of confidentiality, accuracy, and respect. Errors in labeling, testing, or reporting can have irreversible consequences; therefore, attention to detail is not merely procedural but moral. Ethical decision-making also extends to donor recruitment, informed consent, and equitable allocation of blood resources. Professionalism requires lifelong learning, adherence to institutional protocols, and the courage to report discrepancies or unsafe conditions. Through these values, the blood banker embodies the laboratory's highest mission: to ensure that every transfusion is not only scientifically valid but ethically sound.

Chapter 2 - Urinalysis and Body Fluids

Introduction to Urinalysis

Urinalysis represents one of the oldest and most informative diagnostic tools in clinical medicine. The examination of urine provides insight into renal function, metabolic disorders, and systemic disease. Because urine is a filtrate of plasma, it reflects both physiologic and pathologic processes occurring throughout the body. The process of urinalysis typically involves three components: physical, chemical, and microscopic examination. Each offers unique diagnostic value and must be interpreted collectively for clinical relevance. Routine urinalysis is performed not only for symptomatic evaluation but also for screening, monitoring therapeutic progress, and identifying early signs of disease. Technologists must approach every specimen with an understanding of renal physiology, meticulous technique, and careful observation, ensuring that laboratory findings accurately reflect the patient's clinical condition.

Renal Anatomy and Physiology

Accurate interpretation of urinalysis results depends on understanding renal structure and function. Each kidney contains approximately one million nephrons, the microscopic units responsible for filtration, reabsorption, and secretion. Blood enters the glomerulus under pressure, where plasma ultrafiltration occurs, forming the initial filtrate. As this fluid travels through the tubular system—proximal convoluted tubule, loop of Henle, distal tubule, and collecting duct—water, electrolytes, and solutes are selectively reabsorbed or secreted to maintain homeostasis. Hormones such as aldosterone, antidiuretic hormone, and atrial natriuretic peptide finely regulate these processes. The composition of the final urine reflects the kidney's balancing act between waste elimination and conservation of essential substances. Any disruption, whether from glomerular damage, tubular dysfunction, or altered perfusion, manifests as characteristic changes detectable through urinalysis.

Specimen Collection and Handling

The reliability of urinalysis begins with proper specimen collection. Contamination, improper storage, or delayed analysis can alter chemical and microscopic findings. The preferred specimen for routine testing is the first morning urine, as it is most concentrated and reflects overnight renal activity. Midstream clean-catch collection minimizes bacterial contamination and epithelial debris. Once obtained, the specimen should be examined within two hours or refrigerated to prevent bacterial growth and chemical deterioration. Preservation methods, such as chemical additives, are used only when immediate testing is impossible. Technologists must verify identification, labeling, and appearance before analysis. Attention to specimen integrity ensures that results are clinically valid and that patient management decisions are based on accurate laboratory data.

Physical Examination of Urine

The physical characteristics of urine—color, clarity, odor, volume, and specific gravity—offer the first clues to renal and systemic status. Normal urine ranges from pale yellow to amber, reflecting urochrome pigment concentration. Variations in hue may indicate dehydration, hematuria, bilirubinuria, or drug ingestion. Clarity may shift from clear to turbid due to cells, crystals, or microorganisms. Specific gravity, measured by refractometer or reagent strip, reflects the kidney's concentrating ability and hydration status. Foam formation and odor can also provide diagnostic hints; for example, a sweet odor suggests ketosis, while an ammonia-like smell may imply infection. These observations, though simple, guide further testing and underscore the importance of sensory acuity and consistency in laboratory practice.

Chemical Examination of Urine

The chemical analysis, usually performed with reagent strips, screens for key analytes such as protein, glucose, ketones, bilirubin, blood, nitrite, leukocyte esterase, and pH. Each test depends on colorimetric reactions that must be read precisely within specified times. Abnormal findings reveal metabolic or renal disorders: proteinuria may indicate glomerular damage, glucosuria suggests hyperglycemia or renal threshold alteration, and ketonuria points to fat metabolism imbalance. The pH reflects acid-base regulation, while the presence of blood or bilirubin signals pathology requiring correlation with microscopic results. Technologists must interpret chemical reactions in light of specimen handling and interfering substances. The ability to link chemical abnormalities to physiologic mechanisms transforms routine testing into diagnostic insight.

Microscopic Examination

Microscopic evaluation provides direct visualization of formed elements within urine—cells, casts, crystals, bacteria, and other particulates. After centrifugation, the sediment is examined under low and high power. Red blood cells, white blood cells, and epithelial cells indicate inflammation, infection, or trauma. Casts, cylindrical molds formed in renal tubules, signify disease origin within the kidney. Crystals offer metabolic and chemical clues, varying with pH and concentration. Yeast, parasites, and bacteria reveal infectious processes. Mastery of sediment examination requires both technical precision and interpretive skill, integrating morphological patterns with clinical context. The microscopic view serves as the microscope's window into renal health, revealing the stories cells and structures tell about disease.

Examination of Other Body Fluids

Beyond urine, clinical laboratories analyze cerebrospinal, serous, synovial, seminal, and other body fluids. Each specimen type provides distinct diagnostic information while requiring similar analytical principles. Cerebrospinal fluid analysis aids in detecting meningitis or hemorrhage; serous fluids differentiate transudates from exudates; synovial fluid evaluation helps diagnose arthritic disorders. Body fluid analysis emphasizes specimen clarity, viscosity, and cell count, followed by chemical and microbiological assessments. Because these fluids are often collected invasively, sample volume may be limited, demanding prioritization of tests and efficient workflow. Technologists handling body fluids must exercise meticulous care, as results frequently guide urgent clinical interventions and carry significant diagnostic weight.

Clinical Correlation and Disease Patterns

Urinalysis findings gain meaning only when correlated with patient symptoms, medical history, and other laboratory data. The presence of protein and red cells may suggest glomerulonephritis, while glucose and ketones indicate diabetes mellitus. Leukocyte esterase and nitrite positivity together confirm bacterial urinary tract infection. The relationship between laboratory results and clinical manifestations transforms data into diagnosis. Accurate interpretation requires not just memorization but an integrated understanding of pathophysiology. Each abnormality, viewed in context, reveals a chapter of the disease process. Through thoughtful correlation, the medical laboratory technician becomes a translator between microscopic evidence and clinical decision-making.

Automation and Quality Assurance in Urinalysis

Modern urinalysis combines automation with manual verification to achieve efficiency without compromising accuracy. Automated analyzers standardize reagent timing, color reading, and sediment imaging, reducing variability between operators. However, human oversight remains essential for result validation and interpretation of unusual findings. Quality assurance programs monitor reagent integrity, instrument calibration, and technician proficiency. Daily controls confirm accuracy, while documentation provides traceability for audits and accreditation. By integrating technology with vigilance, laboratories ensure consistent reliability. The ultimate goal is a seamless system in which every result, whether automated or manual, reflects truth rather than approximation—a commitment that defines excellence in urinalysis and body fluid testing.

Safety, Ethics, and Professional Conduct

Handling body fluids demands strict adherence to biosafety principles. Universal precautions treat all specimens as potentially infectious, requiring gloves, protective garments, and proper waste disposal. Technologists must balance analytical precision with ethical responsibility, safeguarding patient identity and result confidentiality. Honesty in reporting, verification of anomalies, and refusal to falsify data form the ethical core of laboratory work. Every urine or body fluid sample represents an individual seeking clarity about their health, and respect for that trust defines professional conduct. By uniting safety awareness, technical skill, and ethical integrity, the laboratory professional preserves both the accuracy of results and the dignity of those they serve.

Chapter 3 - Chemistry

Introduction to Clinical Chemistry

Clinical chemistry forms the analytical core of laboratory medicine, translating biochemical processes into measurable data that reflect the physiological and pathological states of the human body. Every test, from glucose estimation to enzyme profiling, measures a dynamic equilibrium between health and disease. The chemical composition of plasma, serum, and other body fluids changes continuously in response to metabolic function, organ performance, and therapeutic intervention. The goal of clinical chemistry is to quantify these changes accurately, enabling clinicians to diagnose conditions, monitor treatment, and prevent complications. To achieve this, medical laboratory technicians must master not only test execution but also the biochemical reasoning behind each measurement. Clinical chemistry unites precision instrumentation, standardized methodology, and interpretive skill to transform chemical reactions into clinical meaning.

Specimen Types and Preanalytical Considerations

The reliability of chemical testing begins before analysis—at the moment of specimen collection. Variations in anticoagulant type, sample handling, and timing can profoundly affect results. Serum is commonly used for chemistry testing, requiring clotting and centrifugation, while plasma allows faster processing but may introduce additive interference. Hemolysis, lipemia, and icterus alter photometric readings, and improper storage degrades labile analytes such as glucose and enzymes. Technicians must observe fasting requirements, label specimens accurately, and maintain temperature control during transport. The preanalytical phase often determines whether data are valid or misleading. Meticulous attention to specimen integrity preserves the connection between patient physiology and the numbers reported on a screen.

Carbohydrate Metabolism and Glucose Testing

Measurement of blood glucose serves as a cornerstone of metabolic assessment. Glucose represents the primary energy substrate for cellular respiration, regulated by hormonal interplay between insulin, glucagon, cortisol, and catecholamines. Persistent elevation indicates diabetes mellitus, while hypoglycemia may reflect insulin excess or metabolic dysfunction. Laboratory testing includes fasting glucose, oral glucose tolerance, and glycated hemoglobin assays. Modern analyzers employ enzymatic methods such as glucose oxidase or hexokinase for specificity and reproducibility. Preanalytical care is crucial, as glycolysis continues in unprocessed samples, lowering measured glucose concentrations. By quantifying carbohydrate metabolism, chemistry testing transforms invisible metabolic imbalance into actionable clinical information, guiding therapeutic adjustment and long-term monitoring.

Protein Analysis and Clinical Significance

Proteins fulfill diverse biological functions—enzymatic catalysis, transport, defense, and structural support. In clinical chemistry, total protein and albumin measurements evaluate nutritional status, hepatic function, and renal integrity. The biuret method remains a standard colorimetric technique, while electrophoresis separates fractions for diagnostic interpretation. Hypoproteinemia may arise from liver disease, nephrotic syndrome, or malnutrition, whereas hyperproteinemia often indicates dehydration or gammopathies. Serum albumin, synthesized by the liver, maintains oncotic pressure and serves as a transport molecule for hormones and drugs. Protein abnormalities often precede overt clinical symptoms, making their detection crucial for early intervention. In the chemistry laboratory, protein analysis exemplifies the union of quantitative precision and biological understanding.

Lipids and Lipoproteins

Lipids play essential roles in cellular structure and energy storage but also contribute to atherosclerosis and cardiovascular disease when dysregulated. Clinical chemistry quantifies cholesterol, triglycerides, and lipoprotein fractions to evaluate metabolic risk. Enzymatic colorimetric methods measure total cholesterol and triglycerides, while high-density and low-density lipoproteins are determined through precipitation or direct assays. Interpretation of lipid panels requires understanding the balance between lipoprotein classes and their influence on vascular health. Fasting specimens minimize chylomicron interference, and results must be correlated with patient history and lifestyle factors. Lipid testing illustrates how chemistry transforms molecular transport into predictive insight, linking biochemical measurement to cardiovascular prevention and management.

Enzymes and Isoenzymes

Enzyme assays occupy a pivotal place in clinical chemistry, providing rapid assessment of tissue damage and metabolic activity. Each enzyme catalyzes a specific reaction, and its presence in serum often signals cell injury. Alanine aminotransferase and aspartate aminotransferase indicate hepatic function, while creatine kinase and lactate dehydrogenase reflect muscle and cardiac integrity. Isoenzyme differentiation enhances diagnostic precision, distinguishing cardiac from skeletal origins. The measurement principle involves monitoring reaction rates through spectrophotometric absorbance, correlating enzymatic velocity with concentration. Technologists must recognize preanalytical influences such as hemolysis and temperature, which alter enzyme stability. Enzymology exemplifies the dynamic relationship between biochemistry and pathology—an ever-changing dialogue recorded by precise measurement.

Electrolytes and Acid-Base Balance

The measurement of electrolytes—sodium, potassium, chloride, and bicarbonate—underpins the evaluation of hydration, renal function, and metabolic balance. Ion-selective electrodes provide rapid, direct quantification, ensuring accuracy in critical care situations. Acid-base interpretation integrates bicarbonate concentration with arterial blood gases to assess respiratory and metabolic disturbances. The relationship between pH, carbon dioxide, and bicarbonate follows the Henderson–Hasselbalch equation, revealing compensatory mechanisms that maintain homeostasis. Errors in electrolyte measurement can mislead therapy, underscoring the necessity for prompt analysis and quality calibration. Through electrolyte and acid-base testing, clinical chemistry captures the body's silent negotiation between acidity and alkalinity, guiding intervention at the biochemical level.

Endocrinology and Hormone Testing

Hormonal assays extend clinical chemistry into the realm of endocrine regulation, encompassing thyroid, adrenal, pituitary, and reproductive hormones. These substances circulate in trace concentrations yet exert profound physiologic control. Modern immunoassay techniques, including enzyme-linked and chemiluminescent methods, detect hormones with extraordinary sensitivity. Interpretation requires awareness of circadian variation, binding proteins, and feedback loops. Thyroid function tests, for example, integrate thyroxine, triiodothyronine, and thyroid-stimulating hormone to evaluate glandular output and pituitary regulation. Endocrine chemistry bridges molecular detection and systemic function, demonstrating how subtle biochemical fluctuations translate into clinical symptoms such as fatigue, weight change, or infertility.

Toxicology and Therapeutic Drug Monitoring

Clinical chemistry also safeguards patient safety through toxicology and therapeutic drug monitoring. Measuring drug and toxin concentrations prevents overdose, ensures compliance, and optimizes therapy. Techniques such as immunoassay screening and confirmatory chromatography identify substances ranging from prescribed medications to environmental poisons. Pharmacokinetics dictate that timing of specimen collection is critical; peak and trough levels must correspond to dosing intervals. Interpretation balances therapeutic effectiveness with avoidance of toxicity. In forensic and emergency contexts, toxicology results often have legal as well as medical consequences. By quantifying substances that heal or harm, the chemistry laboratory functions as both guardian and investigator within healthcare.

Automation, Quality Assurance, and Laboratory Ethics

Automation has transformed chemistry into a discipline of high throughput and precision. Continuous-flow analyzers and modular systems perform hundreds of tests per hour with minimal manual intervention. Despite technological sophistication, human oversight remains central to ensuring data validity. Quality control programs verify calibration, reagent stability, and instrument performance, while proficiency testing demonstrates competence. Ethical practice demands honesty in reporting, critical evaluation of anomalies, and respect for confidentiality. Every result reflects a patient's life, not merely a data point. The true measure of excellence in clinical chemistry lies not only in speed or accuracy but in the unwavering commitment to integrity that defines the laboratory professional.

Download Audio File and Flashcards

Chapter 4 - Hematology

Introduction to Hematology

Hematology encompasses the study of blood, blood-forming organs, and blood diseases. It examines the composition, function, and pathology of the cellular elements—red blood cells, white blood cells, and platelets—within the circulatory system. Through hematologic testing, the laboratory provides crucial insights into oxygen transport, immune response, and hemostasis. Blood analysis extends beyond counting cells; it interprets morphology, biochemical content, and cellular dynamics that reflect systemic health. Each laboratory result forms a narrative of physiologic balance or disturbance. For the medical laboratory technician, hematology represents both an art and a science, demanding precision, interpretive reasoning, and appreciation for the complexity of the human circulatory system.

Hematopoiesis and Bone Marrow Function

The formation of blood cells, or hematopoiesis, occurs primarily in the bone marrow under the influence of growth factors and cytokines. Stem cells within the marrow differentiate into erythroid, myeloid, and megakaryocytic lineages, maintaining a delicate equilibrium between production and destruction. In health, this process ensures adequate cellular renewal; in disease, it may result in cytopenias or proliferative disorders. Bone marrow examination, through aspiration or biopsy, reveals the architecture and activity of hematopoietic tissue. Technologists contribute by preparing and staining smears that display cellular morphology, enabling pathologists to evaluate maturation patterns and detect malignancies. Understanding hematopoiesis anchors the interpretation of peripheral blood findings, linking morphology to marrow physiology.

Erythrocytes and Anemia Evaluation

Red blood cells serve as carriers of oxygen through the hemoglobin molecule, a protein whose structure reflects both genetic design and metabolic regulation. Erythrocyte morphology, size, and hemoglobin content reveal the nature of anemia, one of hematology's most frequent diagnoses. Microcytosis suggests iron deficiency, macrocytosis indicates vitamin B_{12} or folate deficiency, and normocytic anemia may signal chronic disease or blood loss. Laboratory evaluation includes hemoglobin concentration, hematocrit, red cell indices, and reticulocyte count. Peripheral smear examination confirms automated data and identifies abnormal shapes such as spherocytes, target cells, and schistocytes. Through integrated analysis, hematology transforms numeric values into understanding of oxygen-carrying capacity and marrow response.

Hemoglobin and Its Variants

Hemoglobin's role in oxygen transport depends on its iron-heme structure and globin chains. Alterations in these chains give rise to hemoglobinopathies such as sickle cell disease and thalassemia, conditions with profound clinical consequences. Laboratory identification employs electrophoresis, chromatography, or molecular techniques to distinguish variants. Methemoglobin and carboxyhemoglobin testing assess exposure to oxidants and carbon monoxide. Understanding hemoglobin chemistry allows correlation between molecular defects and clinical presentation, from chronic anemia to cyanosis. For the laboratory professional, accurate identification of hemoglobin variants represents both a technical challenge and a crucial contribution to patient management, especially in genetic counseling and transfusion planning.

Leukocytes and Immune Defense

White blood cells form the body's mobile defense system against infection and foreign antigens. The leukocyte differential count quantifies and classifies these cells into neutrophils, lymphocytes, monocytes, eosinophils, and basophils, each with specific immune roles. Neutrophilia typically reflects bacterial infection or inflammation, while lymphocytosis may indicate viral response or lymphoproliferative disease. Morphologic abnormalities, such as toxic granulation or atypical lymphocytes, provide diagnostic clues. Automated counters deliver rapid results, yet microscopic review remains essential to confirm anomalies and detect rare forms such as blasts. Leukocyte evaluation links cellular activity to immune function, transforming microscopic images into evidence of the body's ongoing biological defense.

Platelets and Hemostasis

Platelets, derived from megakaryocytes, are central to primary hemostasis—the process that prevents bleeding following vascular injury. Quantitative and qualitative platelet abnormalities lead to hemorrhagic or thrombotic conditions. Laboratory testing includes platelet count, mean platelet volume, and functional assays such as aggregation studies. Smear evaluation identifies clumping or morphological changes that may explain automated discrepancies. Beyond mechanical clot formation, platelets interact with coagulation factors and endothelium to sustain vascular integrity. The medical laboratory technician ensures the accuracy of platelet data, knowing that each result directly affects clinical decisions regarding transfusion, anticoagulation, or surgery. Hemostasis embodies the balance between bleeding and clotting, a balance the laboratory monitors daily.

Coagulation and Fibrinolysis

The coagulation system comprises a cascade of plasma proteins that culminate in fibrin clot formation. Laboratory assays such as prothrombin time, activated partial thromboplastin time, and fibrinogen concentration evaluate the intrinsic and extrinsic pathways. Abnormal results may indicate factor deficiencies, liver disease, or anticoagulant therapy. Fibrinolysis, the natural process of clot breakdown, is assessed through D-dimer and fibrin degradation product tests. Maintaining standard reagent control and calibration ensures reliability across instruments. In clinical context, coagulation testing guides management of bleeding disorders, thrombosis, and surgical preparation. Mastery of this intricate biochemical network underscores the laboratory's role in sustaining hemostatic equilibrium.

Hematology Instrumentation and Automation

Automation has revolutionized hematology, transforming cell counting and differentiation from manual microscopy to high-speed analysis using electrical impedance and flow cytometry. Automated analyzers generate complete blood counts within seconds, providing indices that reflect red cell size, hemoglobin concentration, and platelet distribution. However, automation complements rather than replaces human evaluation. Abnormal flags prompt smear review, ensuring that unusual morphology or artifacts are identified. Calibration, maintenance, and quality control uphold instrument accuracy. Automation enables laboratories to process high volumes efficiently, yet interpretation and correlation remain the professional's domain. The blend of technology and human expertise defines modern hematologic practice.

Quality Assurance and Error Prevention

Every hematologic result must be defensible, reproducible, and clinically sound. Quality assurance programs monitor analytical precision through internal controls, external proficiency testing, and instrument performance verification. Preanalytical factors such as anticoagulant ratio, sample mixing, and storage can distort results if neglected. Technologists bear responsibility for recognizing inconsistencies, verifying flagged results, and documenting corrective actions. Peer review, reagent validation, and statistical control charts maintain ongoing accuracy. Through these practices, hematology exemplifies the laboratory's commitment to evidence-based reliability. The patient's well-being depends on data integrity, and quality assurance transforms that obligation into daily discipline.

Safety, Ethics, and Professional Integrity

Hematology laboratories handle biohazardous materials, sharps, and infectious samples, requiring adherence to safety protocols and regulatory standards. Personal protective equipment, proper waste disposal, and awareness of bloodborne pathogen precautions form the basis of safe practice. Beyond technical skill, ethical integrity governs result reporting and patient confidentiality. The hematology professional must avoid bias, acknowledge uncertainty, and communicate findings transparently. Each blood specimen carries both scientific and human value—it represents a life requiring precise interpretation. Through ethical conduct, continuous education, and respect for the profession's standards, the medical laboratory technician preserves the trust placed in laboratory medicine.

Chapter 5 - Immunology

Foundations of Immunology

Immunology is the study of the body's defense mechanisms against foreign substances. It explores how cells and molecules recognize, respond to, and eliminate potential threats. The immune system functions through innate and adaptive components that operate in harmony to maintain internal equilibrium. Innate immunity provides rapid, nonspecific protection through physical barriers, phagocytes, and complement proteins, while adaptive immunity confers specific recognition and memory via lymphocytes. The laboratory's role in immunology is to measure, interpret, and apply these biological responses for diagnosis and monitoring. Through precise testing, technologists translate cellular and molecular reactions into clinical understanding, linking invisible immune processes to visible laboratory data that guide patient care.

Cells and Organs of the Immune System

The cellular architecture of the immune system is distributed throughout specialized tissues and organs. Bone marrow serves as the origin of all blood cells, including lymphocytes, which mature into B cells in the marrow and T cells in the thymus. These lymphocytes populate secondary lymphoid organs such as the spleen, lymph nodes, and mucosa-associated lymphoid tissue, where antigen encounter initiates immune activation. Macrophages, dendritic cells, and natural killer cells provide surveillance and initial defense. The coordination among these cells ensures that pathogens are identified, neutralized, and remembered for future protection. Understanding this organization allows the medical laboratory technician to interpret test results within the physiological context of immune function.

Antigens and Antibodies

Antigens are molecular structures capable of eliciting an immune response, whereas antibodies are the proteins produced by B lymphocytes in response. Each antibody recognizes a specific antigenic determinant, forming a lock-and-key interaction that defines immune specificity. Antibodies consist of two heavy and two light chains forming variable regions for antigen binding and constant regions that mediate effector functions such as complement activation. Laboratory assays exploit these interactions to detect infection, autoimmune disease, and immunodeficiency. The strength and type of antibody response—IgM for early reaction, IgG for long-term immunity—carry diagnostic significance. By understanding antigen–antibody relationships, technologists convert immunologic principles into measurable outcomes.

The Complement System

The complement system is a cascade of plasma proteins that amplifies immune responses, leading to pathogen lysis, inflammation, and phagocytosis. Activation occurs through classical, alternative, or lectin pathways, all converging at the cleavage of C3. The resulting fragments promote opsonization, chemotaxis, and membrane attack complex formation. Complement deficiencies predispose individuals to recurrent infections or autoimmune disorders, while overactivation contributes to tissue damage in inflammatory diseases. Laboratory tests such as total hemolytic complement (CH_{50}) and component-specific assays evaluate functional integrity. Recognizing complement activity allows correlation between immunologic mechanism and clinical manifestation, reinforcing the technician's role in translating complex biochemical cascades into meaningful diagnostic insight.

Immune Response and Hypersensitivity

The immune response encompasses activation, proliferation, and regulation of lymphocytes following antigen exposure. Ideally, this reaction protects the host without causing harm; however, hypersensitivity arises when the response becomes exaggerated or misdirected. Four major types are recognized: immediate (Type I), cytotoxic (Type II), immune complex (Type III), and delayed-type (Type IV). Each involves distinct mechanisms ranging from IgE-mediated allergic reactions to T-cell-driven inflammation. Laboratory detection of specific antibodies, immune complexes, or cytokine profiles assists in identifying hypersensitivity disorders. Understanding these mechanisms not only clarifies disease pathology but also underscores the fine balance between defense and self-damage that defines immunologic health.

Autoimmunity and Immune Tolerance

Immune tolerance prevents the body from attacking its own tissues, a balance maintained through deletion or inactivation of self-reactive lymphocytes. When this control fails, autoimmunity develops, producing chronic inflammatory diseases such as systemic lupus erythematosus or rheumatoid arthritis. The laboratory's role involves detecting autoantibodies against nuclear, cytoplasmic, or organ-specific antigens using immunofluorescence, enzyme-linked, or agglutination methods. Positive findings must be interpreted alongside clinical symptoms, as autoantibodies may precede or persist without disease. Understanding tolerance mechanisms and autoimmune triggers enables laboratory professionals to assist in early detection and monitoring of these conditions, providing clinicians with data essential for targeted therapy and prognosis.

Immunodeficiency Disorders

Defects in immune development or function lead to immunodeficiency, characterized by increased susceptibility to infection. Primary immunodeficiencies are congenital, such as severe combined immunodeficiency or IgA deficiency, whereas secondary causes include malnutrition, malignancy, and immunosuppressive therapy. Laboratory evaluation includes measurement of immunoglobulin levels, lymphocyte subsets, and functional assays of neutrophil and complement activity. Early identification of immune deficits is critical for preventing recurrent or severe infections. Technologists play an essential role in recognizing abnormal results that suggest impaired immunity and ensuring quality control in these highly specialized tests. Immunodeficiency testing merges diagnostic precision with profound clinical impact, reflecting the laboratory's central contribution to patient management.

Serological Testing and Diagnostic Applications

Serology applies immunologic principles to detect antibodies or antigens in patient samples. Tests such as agglutination, precipitation, enzyme-linked immunosorbent assay, and chemiluminescence are fundamental tools for diagnosing infectious diseases and immune disorders. The choice of method depends on desired sensitivity, specificity, and turnaround time. Accurate serologic testing requires strict quality control, appropriate sample selection, and correlation with clinical findings. In infectious disease monitoring, rising antibody titers signify active infection or recent exposure, whereas persistent IgG suggests past immunity. By mastering serological techniques, medical laboratory technicians convert immunologic reactions into precise diagnostic evidence that directs clinical decisions and epidemiologic surveillance.

Molecular Immunology and Advanced Techniques

Modern immunology increasingly incorporates molecular technology to characterize immune components at the genetic level. Polymerase chain reaction and flow cytometry allow quantification of cell populations, gene expression, and cytokine production. These methods identify clonal expansions in lymphoid malignancies and detect minimal residual disease. Flow cytometry, in particular, revolutionized immunophenotyping by using fluorescently labeled antibodies to define cell surface markers with exquisite precision. Molecular immunology extends traditional serology into genomic and proteomic dimensions, revealing mechanisms underlying immune regulation and dysfunction. As these technologies evolve, laboratory professionals must continually update their knowledge, integrating molecular data with classical immunologic interpretation to deliver comprehensive diagnostic insight.

Quality Assurance and Professional Practice in Immunology

Immunologic testing demands rigorous attention to detail and adherence to quality standards. Variability in reagents, incubation times, and environmental conditions can alter outcomes. Regular calibration, control materials, and participation in external proficiency programs maintain reliability. Ethical responsibility requires transparency in reporting limitations and awareness of cross-reactivity or false positives. Confidentiality of patient data and respect for biosafety are paramount. The immunology professional bridges analytical skill with ethical integrity, ensuring that each reported result reflects scientific accuracy and moral responsibility. Through continual education and quality assurance, immunology laboratories uphold the trust placed in diagnostic medicine and sustain the credibility of clinical science.

Chapter 6 - Microbiology

Introduction to Microbiology

Microbiology examines the microscopic world of organisms—bacteria, viruses, fungi, and parasites—that influence human health. In clinical practice, it forms the foundation of infection diagnosis, antimicrobial management, and public health surveillance. The medical laboratory technician serves as both investigator and guardian, identifying pathogens that may threaten individual or community wellbeing. Modern microbiology blends classical culture methods with molecular diagnostics to detect even minute traces of microorganisms. Each test result carries implications for treatment, infection control, and epidemiology. Microbiology thus functions not as an isolated discipline but as the connecting thread linking laboratory science, clinical medicine, and patient recovery.

Specimen Collection and Processing

Accurate microbiological results depend primarily on proper specimen collection and timely processing. Each type of infection requires a specific sample—blood for bacteremia, sputum for respiratory infection, or cerebrospinal fluid for meningitis. Contamination during collection can obscure true pathogens, leading to diagnostic error. Specimens must be labeled precisely, transported promptly, and maintained under appropriate temperature conditions. Upon arrival in the laboratory, they are logged, inoculated onto suitable media, and incubated under defined atmospheric environments. The technologist must judge specimen quality, as poor collection invalidates even the most sophisticated testing. Proper handling at every step ensures that microbial isolation reflects the patient's true infectious state rather than procedural artifact.

Culture Media and Growth Requirements

Culture media serve as the lifeblood of microbiology, providing nutrients and conditions necessary for microbial growth. Basic media such as nutrient agar support nonfastidious organisms, while enriched formulations like blood or chocolate agar enable recovery of delicate pathogens. Selective and differential media incorporate inhibitors and indicators to isolate specific groups, such as MacConkey agar for enteric Gram-negative bacilli. Temperature, pH, oxygen concentration, and moisture each influence growth. The technologist must understand these requirements to cultivate pathogens successfully and recognize contamination. Mastery of media selection transforms a Petri dish into a diagnostic tool, revealing invisible infections through visible colonies that guide treatment decisions.

Bacteriology and Identification Methods

Bacteriology forms the core of clinical microbiology, encompassing isolation, identification, and antimicrobial susceptibility testing of bacterial pathogens. Gram staining provides the initial differentiation, followed by biochemical profiling through catalase, oxidase, and carbohydrate fermentation reactions. Automated identification systems and matrix-assisted laser desorption ionization mass spectrometry (MALDI-TOF) now accelerate organism recognition with remarkable precision. Still, interpretation requires human discernment—colony morphology, hemolytic pattern, and odor remain valuable diagnostic clues. Accurate identification determines therapy, infection control measures, and public health reporting. Each culture plate represents a clinical mystery unraveled by the technologist's careful observation and scientific reasoning.

Antimicrobial Susceptibility Testing

Determining a microorganism's response to antimicrobial agents is essential for effective therapy. Susceptibility testing, performed by disk diffusion, broth dilution, or automated systems, quantifies the minimal inhibitory concentration required to suppress growth. Results are interpreted according to standardized guidelines, categorizing isolates as susceptible, intermediate, or resistant. These data guide clinicians in antibiotic selection and track emerging resistance trends. Quality control organisms ensure test validity, while error in interpretation can compromise patient care. The laboratory's vigilance in monitoring resistance supports the global fight against antimicrobial misuse and evolving pathogens. In this balance between therapy and resistance, the microbiology laboratory serves as a sentinel for modern medicine.

Mycology and Fungal Identification

Mycology addresses the diverse world of yeasts and molds that cause opportunistic and systemic infections. While most fungi are harmless environmental organisms, certain species—such as Candida, Aspergillus, and Cryptococcus—pose significant threats to immunocompromised patients. Diagnosis depends on culture, microscopy, and increasingly, antigen and molecular detection. Fungal colonies require prolonged incubation and specialized media, making patience a vital skill in mycology. Microscopic identification relies on recognizing hyphal structure, spore formation, and pigment production. The medical laboratory technician must correlate culture results with clinical presentation, as colonization and infection often overlap. Fungal diagnosis exemplifies the delicate intersection between environmental exposure and host susceptibility.

Parasitology and Identification of Protozoa and Helminths

Parasitology explores organisms that depend on human hosts for survival and reproduction. Protozoa and helminths cause diseases with global significance, including malaria, giardiasis, and schistosomiasis. Laboratory detection involves microscopic examination of stool, blood, or tissue specimens using concentration techniques and permanent stains. Recognition of motility, morphology, and life cycle stages requires extensive training and keen observation. Rapid antigen and molecular tests now complement microscopy, improving detection where parasite loads are low. Parasitology teaches patience and precision—each field of view under the microscope may hold the single organism that confirms diagnosis. The technologist's expertise ensures that parasitic diseases, often overlooked, receive timely and accurate identification.

Virology and Molecular Detection

Viruses, though among the smallest infectious agents, exert enormous clinical and epidemiological impact. Virology focuses on identifying these obligate intracellular pathogens through culture, antigen detection, serology, and molecular amplification. Cell culture remains valuable for some viruses, but polymerase chain reaction (PCR) and next-generation sequencing now dominate due to speed and sensitivity. Quantitative viral load testing guides treatment in chronic infections such as HIV and hepatitis. The laboratory's role in virology extends beyond diagnosis—it contributes to outbreak surveillance, vaccine evaluation, and epidemiologic research. Each viral genome analyzed adds to collective understanding, transforming molecular sequences into meaningful clinical insight.

Infection Control and Public Health Microbiology

Microbiology extends beyond individual patients into the realm of community health. The laboratory monitors hospital-acquired infections, tracks resistant organisms, and collaborates with infection control teams to contain outbreaks. Surveillance cultures, environmental sampling, and molecular typing identify transmission pathways. Adherence to biosafety levels and proper decontamination protocols protects laboratory personnel and prevents cross-contamination. The integration of microbiology into public health ensures early detection of emerging pathogens and supports national reporting systems. In every result reported, the technologist participates in safeguarding not just one life but the health of populations—a reminder that microbiology is both scientific pursuit and civic duty.

Quality Assurance, Biosafety, and Professional Ethics

The precision of microbiological diagnosis relies on stringent quality assurance and adherence to biosafety standards. Regular monitoring of media performance, reagent sterility, and instrument calibration ensures validity. Biosafety practices, including appropriate containment, personal protective equipment, and waste management, protect laboratory staff from infection. Ethical conduct demands accurate reporting, avoidance of data manipulation, and respect for confidentiality. Errors in microbiology can have far-reaching consequences, from misdiagnosis to epidemic spread. The professional integrity of the microbiologist lies in steadfast commitment to accuracy, safety, and honesty. In every culture plate and molecular assay, ethical practice sustains the credibility of science and the trust of society

Chapter 7 - Laboratory Operations

Foundations of Laboratory Management

Laboratory operations form the framework that sustains every aspect of clinical testing. Management integrates personnel, instrumentation, workflow, and quality systems to ensure accurate and timely results. Effective laboratory leadership requires both technical knowledge and administrative skill. Each test performed represents a coordinated effort between specimen collection, analytical processing, and result interpretation. Standard operating procedures, documentation, and communication channels establish order within this complex environment. Laboratory management also addresses budgeting, inventory control, and strategic planning. A well-managed laboratory operates not by chance but by design, transforming technical precision into consistent service excellence that supports patient care and institutional goals.

Quality Assurance and Quality Control

Quality assurance encompasses the entire testing process—preanalytical, analytical, and postanalytical—while quality control verifies daily performance within that framework. Together they form the foundation of laboratory reliability. Control materials with known values are tested alongside patient samples to confirm instrument accuracy and reagent stability. Results are evaluated statistically, with corrective action initiated for deviations. Quality assurance extends further, monitoring specimen handling, documentation, and reporting accuracy. Accreditation agencies require continuous review of performance indicators and participation in proficiency testing. The medical laboratory technician's vigilance in quality control ensures that every result released represents scientific truth, maintaining the laboratory's integrity and the clinician's trust.

Laboratory Safety and Risk Management

Safety in the laboratory protects personnel, patients, and the environment from biological, chemical, and physical hazards. Risk management begins with hazard identification, training, and strict adherence to universal precautions. Biosafety levels dictate containment procedures based on pathogen risk, while chemical hygiene plans govern reagent handling and waste disposal. Emergency preparedness includes spill control, fire prevention, and first aid response. Technicians must also recognize ergonomic and radiation risks within the laboratory setting. A culture of safety transforms compliance into habit, where every task is performed with awareness and respect for potential danger. By prioritizing safety, the laboratory affirms that human wellbeing outweighs operational speed or convenience.

Laboratory Mathematics and Instrumentation

Mathematical competence underpins all quantitative laboratory work. Technologists perform calculations for dilutions, concentrations, conversion factors, and quality control statistics. Understanding significant figures, standard deviation, and coefficient of variation ensures accurate interpretation of numerical data. Instrumentation integrates these mathematical concepts with analytical technology—spectrophotometry, automation, and data processing. Calibration curves translate absorbance into concentration, while maintenance logs verify consistent performance. A single miscalculation can distort results, emphasizing the importance of precision and verification. Mathematics and instrumentation together represent the language and logic of laboratory science, where each number, formula, and calibration point contributes to diagnostic certainty.

Regulatory Compliance and Accreditation

Clinical laboratories operate under rigorous regulatory oversight designed to ensure public safety and data validity. Agencies such as the Clinical Laboratory Improvement Amendments (CLIA), the College of American Pathologists (CAP), and The Joint Commission establish standards for personnel qualifications, quality systems, and proficiency testing. Compliance audits evaluate adherence to these standards, and deficiencies require documented corrective actions. Accreditation not only validates technical competence but also demonstrates ethical accountability. The medical laboratory technician contributes by maintaining accurate records, following procedures, and preparing for inspections. Regulatory compliance embodies the laboratory's ethical contract with society: to deliver results that are accurate, traceable, and defensible.

Information Management and Laboratory Informatics

The digital age has transformed laboratory operations through informatics systems that manage data from specimen accessioning to result reporting. Laboratory Information Systems (LIS) integrate analyzers, middleware, and hospital databases to reduce manual entry errors and accelerate workflow. Technologists must understand data verification, system security, and confidentiality protocols under privacy regulations. Informatics also supports quality improvement through analytics and trend monitoring. As automation increases, human oversight ensures that data integrity remains uncompromised. Information management is not merely technological—it is ethical stewardship of medical information, demanding accuracy, confidentiality, and accountability at every keystroke.

Communication and Interpersonal Skills

Effective communication links the laboratory to clinicians, nurses, and patients. Technologists must convey results clearly, document findings accurately, and respond professionally to inquiries or critical values. Within the laboratory, teamwork depends on mutual respect and precise verbal and written exchange. Miscommunication can delay diagnosis or compromise patient safety. Emotional intelligence, cultural awareness, and active listening strengthen collaboration in multidisciplinary healthcare environments. The laboratory professional's communication style reflects competence and reliability, ensuring that the science within the laboratory translates into understanding at the bedside. Clear communication transforms technical data into actionable medical information.

Inventory Control and Equipment Maintenance

Operational efficiency relies on consistent supply availability and properly functioning instruments. Inventory control involves forecasting reagent usage, monitoring expiration dates, and preventing waste through systematic ordering. Equipment maintenance ensures accuracy and longevity; daily checks, calibration, and preventive servicing prevent downtime and costly repairs. Documentation of maintenance activity satisfies accreditation requirements and demonstrates accountability. The medical laboratory technician's attention to equipment and supply details supports uninterrupted testing and financial responsibility. Through careful stewardship of resources, the laboratory transforms routine maintenance into a culture of reliability and fiscal prudence.

Ethics, Professionalism, and Confidentiality

Ethical conduct is the cornerstone of laboratory operations. Professionals must perform duties with honesty, respect, and impartiality, ensuring that every action upholds patient welfare. Confidentiality protects individuals' privacy, while professionalism ensures respectful interaction and accountability. Breach of ethics—whether data falsification, unauthorized disclosure, or negligence—undermines the credibility of the laboratory and the entire healthcare system. Continuous education, adherence to institutional policies, and awareness of legal responsibilities strengthen ethical competence. Professionalism extends beyond technical skill to moral integrity, defining the laboratory technician not merely as a worker but as a custodian of trust within medicine.

Continuous Improvement and Leadership Development

A successful laboratory evolves through continuous improvement—systematic evaluation, innovation, and staff development. Regular audits, root cause analyses, and performance metrics identify opportunities for enhancement. Leadership development encourages technologists to contribute ideas, mentor peers, and assume responsibility for quality outcomes. Continuing education ensures readiness for technological and regulatory changes. The pursuit of excellence becomes a shared mission, uniting staff around the goal of superior patient care. In cultivating leadership and improvement, the laboratory transforms from a static testing center into a dynamic institution of learning, growth, and professional pride that embodies the future of clinical science.

Chapter 8 – Practice Questions

Question (1-100)

Q1. Which of the following antigens is most immunogenic within the Rh blood group system?

(A) c

(B) D

(C) E

(D) C

Q2. A blood donor's sample shows a positive anti-D antibody screen. What is the most likely cause?

(A) Autoimmune disease

(B) Exposure to cold

(C) Recent vaccination

(D) Rh immunization

Q3. The universal donor for packed red blood cells is:

(A) AB positive

(B) O negative

(C) O positive

(D) AB negative

Q4. Which antibody class is responsible for hemolytic disease of the newborn (HDN)?

(A) IgG

(B) IgD

(C) IgA

(D) IgM

Q5. Which temperature range best supports optimal reactivity for IgM antibodies in blood banking tests?

(A) 37°C

(B) 4°C

(C) 56°C

(D) 22°C

Q6. Which antigen system is enhanced by enzyme treatment of red blood cells?

(A) Kell

(B) Rh

(C) Duffy

(D) MNS

Q7. A positive direct antiglobulin test (DAT) indicates:

(A) Presence of circulating antibodies

(B) Autoimmune liver disease

(C) Antibodies attached to red cells in vivo

(D) Complement binding to plasma proteins

Q8. The antiglobulin reagent used in the Coombs test contains:

(A) Complement C5 fragments

(B) Anti-human IgG and anti-C3

(C) Only anti-IgA

(D) Saline and albumin only

Q9. Which blood group antigen is associated with protection against Plasmodium vivax infection?

(A) Kell

(B) Duffy

(C) Kidd

(D) MNS

Q10. Which antibody type typically causes delayed hemolytic transfusion reactions?

(A) Cold autoantibody
(B) Complement-fixing IgM
(C) Alloimmune IgG
(D) Naturally occurring IgM

Q11. Which of the following methods confirms ABO grouping discrepancies?

(A) DAT
(B) Saline replacement technique
(C) Secretor testing
(D) Enzyme treatment

Q12. The weak D test is performed to detect:

(A) Cold autoantibody
(B) Partial D variant
(C) Missing Rh antigen
(D) Anti-E reactivity

Q13. Which additive prevents complement activation in plasma used for antibody screening?

(A) EDTA
(B) Sodium fluoride
(C) Heparin
(D) Sodium citrate

Q14. An AB-negative individual has which antibodies in plasma?

(A) Anti-A
(B) Anti-B and anti-D
(C) Anti-A and anti-B
(D) None

Q15. In routine compatibility testing, the major crossmatch detects:

(A) Donor and recipient cells mixed in saline
(B) Complement activation in donor plasma
(C) Donor serum against recipient cells
(D) Donor cells against recipient serum

Q16. A patient develops chills and fever six hours post-transfusion without hemolysis. What is the most probable cause?

(A) Febrile non-hemolytic reaction
(B) Allergic reaction
(C) Acute hemolysis
(D) Bacterial contamination

Q17. RhIG administration prevents sensitization by:

(A) Inducing complement fixation
(B) Coating fetal cells for clearance
(C) Blocking antigen presentation
(D) Stimulating IgG production

Q18. Which antigen group is destroyed by enzymes during testing?

(A) Kell
(B) Kidd
(C) Rh
(D) Duffy

Q19. Which reagent is essential for the indirect antiglobulin test (IAT)?

(A) Polyspecific Coombs reagent
(B) Anti-A lectin
(C) Bromelin enzyme
(D) Saline control

Q20. Which condition causes a false-negative antiglobulin test?
(A) Use of old serum
(B) Excess washing
(C) Inadequate washing
(D) Overcentrifugation

Q21. Which of the following antibodies is clinically insignificant in transfusion testing?
(A) Anti-K
(B) Anti-Jka
(C) Anti-D
(D) Anti-I

Q22. Which technique is used for antibody elution from sensitized red cells?
(A) Adsorption
(B) Enzyme-linked assay
(C) Gel filtration
(D) Heat or acid elution

Q23. The Kell antigen system is significant because:
(A) It is IgM-reactive
(B) It occurs only in neonates
(C) It causes mild hemolysis
(D) It resists enzyme destruction

Q24. Which antibody causes severe immediate hemolytic transfusion reaction?
(A) Anti-M
(B) Anti-Jka
(C) Anti-A
(D) Anti-Lea

Q25. A Kell-negative woman should not receive Kell-positive blood because:
(A) It triggers autoantibody formation
(B) It produces anti-K alloantibodies
(C) It increases viscosity
(D) It affects iron metabolism

Q26. Which test differentiates autoantibody from alloantibody in a patient's serum?
(A) Forward grouping
(B) Direct antiglobulin test
(C) Adsorption studies
(D) Saline replacement method

Q27. Which antibody screening phase detects clinically significant IgG antibodies?
(A) Immediate spin (room temperature)
(B) Complement fixation
(C) 37 °C incubation and AHG phase
(D) 4 °C saline test

Q28. What is the function of low-ionic-strength saline (LISS) in antibody detection?
(A) Remove bound IgG
(B) Reduce ionic strength to accelerate binding
(C) Increase RBC zeta potential

(D) Destroy complement proteins

Q29. An Rh-negative woman delivers an Rh-positive baby. What test determines fetal maternal hemorrhage volume?

(A) Indirect Coombs test
(B) Rosette screen
(C) Kleihauer-Betke test
(D) Direct Coombs test

Q30. Which antibody most frequently causes delayed hemolytic transfusion reactions?

(A) Anti-K
(B) Anti-E
(C) Anti-Lea
(D) Anti-Jka

Q31. Which antigen system exhibits dosage effect most strongly?

(A) Duffy
(B) Lewis
(C) P
(D) ABO

Q32. What is the storage temperature for red blood cell units?

(A) 1-6 °C
(B) -18 °C
(C) 20-24 °C
(D) -65 °C

Q33. Which situation requires issuing irradiated blood components?

(A) Iron deficiency
(B) Congenital immunodeficiency
(C) Severe anemia
(D) Autoimmune hemolysis

Q34. Which plasma component provides the highest fibrinogen concentration?

(A) Platelet concentrate
(B) Fresh Frozen Plasma
(C) Cryoprecipitate
(D) Albumin solution

Q35. During transfusion, the patient develops back pain and hemoglobinuria within minutes. What should be done first?

(A) Stop transfusion immediately
(B) Notify blood bank after completion
(C) Continue transfusion at slower rate
(D) Add saline to the unit

Q36. Which blood group antigen is resistant to enzyme treatment?

(A) N
(B) Duffy
(C) Kell
(D) M

Q37. Which screening test detects unexpected antibodies in patient plasma before transfusion?

(A) Typing for ABO only
(B) Crossmatch
(C) Antibody screen
(D) Direct Coombs

Q38. Which of the following can cause a false-positive antiglobulin test?
(A) Overwashing of cells
(B) Dirty glassware
(C) Inadequate centrifugation
(D) Cold agglutinins
Q39. Which of the following is the universal plasma donor type?
(A) O
(B) AB
(C) A
(D) B
Q40. A unit of whole blood has been stored for 30 days. Which change is expected?
(A) Decreased potassium
(B) Decreased 2,3-DPG and pH
(C) Increased glucose
(D) Increased pH
Q41. Which antibody demonstrates complement activation leading to intravascular hemolysis?
(A) Anti-A
(B) Anti-Fya
(C) Anti-D
(D) Anti-K
Q42. What is the primary function of the antiglobulin test in transfusion medicine?
(A) Measure plasma proteins
(B) Determine hematocrit
(C) Detect sensitized RBCs
(D) Detect unbound antibody
Q43. Which antigen is found on the majority of Rh-positive individuals?
(A) e
(B) D
(C) C
(D) c
Q44. Which additive extends red-cell shelf life to 42 days?
(A) CPDA-1
(B) AS-1 (Adsol)
(C) ACD-A
(D) CPD
Q45. What is the maximum storage time for platelets at 20-24 °C with agitation?
(A) 3 days
(B) 5 days
(C) 35 days
(D) 21 days
Q46. Which plasma factor is most labile and requires rapid freezing of FFP?
(A) Factor X
(B) Factor II
(C) Factor V
(D) Factor VII
Q47. Which ABO group is known as the universal recipient for RBC transfusion?
(A) O positive
(B) AB positive

(C) A positive
(D) B positive
Q48. Which blood product is indicated for a patient with thrombotic thrombocytopenic purpura (TTP)?
(A) Cryoprecipitate
(B) Packed RBCs
(C) Platelets
(D) Plasma exchange (FFP)
Q49. Which quality-control parameter must be checked daily in blood bank refrigerators?
(A) Humidity
(B) Temperature recording
(C) Light intensity
(D) pH
Q50. Which of the following antibodies is most commonly associated with HDN after anti-D?
(A) Anti-Lea
(B) Anti-N
(C) Anti-Jkb
(D) Anti-K
Q51. Which of the following conditions requires washed red blood cells for transfusion?
(A) Febrile non-hemolytic transfusion reaction
(B) Iron deficiency anemia
(C) Severe allergic reaction to plasma proteins
(D) Mild anemia with low hemoglobin
Q52. Which antibody is most commonly associated with paroxysmal cold hemoglobinuria (PCH)?
(A) Anti-D
(B) Anti-P
(C) Anti-Lea
(D) Anti-I
Q53. Which technique is most appropriate for antibody identification when multiple antibodies are suspected?
(A) Saline crossmatch
(B) Enzyme panel
(C) Antibody panel with selected cells
(D) Forward typing
Q54. What type of antibody is Anti-A1, occasionally found in A2 individuals?
(A) Alloimmune IgG
(B) Complement-dependent IgG
(C) Naturally occurring IgM
(D) IgA cold-reactive
Q55. In which of the following conditions would autoadsorption NOT be appropriate?
(A) Recently transfused patient
(B) Warm autoimmune hemolytic anemia
(C) Drug-induced immune hemolysis
(D) Cold agglutinin disease
Q56. Which antibody enhancement reagent works by lowering zeta potential and promoting RBC sensitization?
(A) Enzyme (papain)
(B) LISS

(C) Albumin
(D) PEG
Q57. Which of the following reactions is most severe in ABO-incompatible transfusions?
(A) Delayed extravascular hemolysis
(B) Acute intravascular hemolysis
(C) Urticarial reaction
(D) Febrile reaction
Q58. Which antigen system is located on glycophorin A and B of the red cell membrane?
(A) Duffy
(B) Kell
(C) Kidd
(D) MNS
Q59. What is the maximum shelf life for frozen RBCs stored at -65 °C or colder?
(A) 10 years
(B) 5 years
(C) 1 year
(D) 90 days
Q60. Which condition is best prevented by Rh immune globulin (RhIG)?
(A) Febrile transfusion reaction
(B) Transfusion-associated GVHD
(C) Rh sensitization and HDN
(D) ABO incompatibility
Q61. The Rh-null phenotype lacks which of the following?
(A) E and e antigens only
(B) D antigen only
(C) All Rh system antigens
(D) C and c antigens only
Q62. Which step in transfusion testing ensures patient identity verification before blood issue?
(A) ABO typing
(B) Crossmatch
(C) Clerical check
(D) Antibody screen
Q63. Which component should be transfused to a patient with isolated factor VIII deficiency?
(A) Whole blood
(B) FFP
(C) Cryoprecipitate
(D) Platelets
Q64. Which antibody is most likely to show enhanced reactivity after enzyme treatment?
(A) Anti-Fya
(B) Anti-M
(C) Anti-Jka
(D) Anti-S
Q65. A mixed-field agglutination pattern in forward ABO typing indicates:
(A) Recent transfusion or bone marrow transplant
(B) Weak subgroup of A
(C) Polyagglutination
(D) Cold autoantibody interference
Q66. Which test differentiates true hemolytic disease from passive antibody transfer?

(A) DAT only
(B) Elution and antibody identification
(C) Rosette test
(D) Indirect Coombs

Q67. In the Lewis system, which phenotype is typical of cord blood?
(A) Le(a+b+)
(B) Le(a-b+)
(C) Le(a+b-)
(D) Le(a-b-)

Q68. Which substance can neutralize certain antibodies such as Anti-Lea during testing?
(A) Saliva from secretor individuals
(B) Enzymes
(C) Ficin-treated RBCs
(D) Albumin reagent

Q69. Which blood product is indicated for neonatal exchange transfusion?
(A) Random platelet concentrate
(B) Whole blood from any donor
(C) Group O, Rh-negative, irradiated, CMV-negative RBCs
(D) Group AB, Rh-positive plasma

Q70. Which storage lesion in RBCs most affects oxygen delivery?
(A) Decreased 2,3-DPG
(B) Increased potassium
(C) Decreased ATP
(D) Hemolysis

Q71. Which hormone primarily regulates water reabsorption in the distal nephron?
(A) Antidiuretic hormone (ADH)
(B) Aldosterone
(C) Atrial natriuretic peptide (ANP)
(D) Renin

Q72. A urine specimen has a specific gravity of 1.035. Which interpretation is most accurate?
(A) Normal concentrating ability
(B) Dilute urine sample
(C) Renal concentrating failure
(D) Possible radiographic dye contamination

Q73. Which of the following would produce a false-positive protein result on a reagent strip test?
(A) Acidic urine pH
(B) Elevated glucose concentration
(C) Highly alkaline urine
(D) Ascorbic acid presence

Q74. A refrigerated urine sample left at room temperature for several hours will likely show:
(A) Increased bacteria and nitrite
(B) Stable glucose and ketones
(C) Increased WBC integrity
(D) Decreased pH and odor

Q75. Which urinary structure functions primarily in filtration of plasma?
(A) Loop of Henle
(B) Glomerulus
(C) Distal convoluted tubule

(D) Collecting duct

Q76. A red, hazy urine with a positive dipstick for blood but no RBCs microscopically suggests:

(A) Bacterial infection

(B) Hematuria

(C) Myoglobinuria

(D) Menstrual contamination

Q77. Which reagent strip test detects glucose via the glucose oxidase reaction?

(A) Ketone (nitroprusside) test

(B) Glucose oxidase-peroxidase color reaction

(C) Clinitest tablet method

(D) Copper reduction test

Q78. Presence of RBC casts in urine sediment signifies:

(A) Renal glomerular damage

(B) Bacterial cystitis

(C) Vaginal contamination

(D) Lower urinary tract bleeding

Q79. Which urinary crystal is hexagonal and seen in cystinuria?

(A) Leucine

(B) Tyrosine

(C) Cystine

(D) Cholesterol

Q80. What is the normal range of cerebrospinal fluid (CSF) glucose relative to plasma?

(A) About 2/3 of plasma glucose

(B) Equal to plasma glucose

(C) 50% higher than plasma glucose

(D) Unrelated to plasma glucose

Q81. In which condition is urine specific gravity fixed around 1.010, regardless of fluid intake?

(A) Diabetes insipidus

(B) Dehydration

(C) Diabetes mellitus

(D) Chronic renal failure (isosthenuria)

Q82. The presence of white blood cell casts indicates:

(A) Lower urinary tract infection

(B) Glomerular bleeding

(C) Pyelonephritis or interstitial nephritis

(D) Tubular necrosis

Q83. Which component is responsible for the gel matrix of urinary casts?

(A) Hemoglobin

(B) Tamm-Horsfall protein

(C) Myoglobin

(D) Albumin

Q84. Which test confirms reducing substances other than glucose in urine?

(A) Ictotest tablet test

(B) Clinitest (copper reduction)

(C) Reagent strip glucose test

(D) Acetest ketone test

Q85. A milky urine that clears after adding acetic acid suggests:

(A) Chyluria

(B) Phosphaturia
(C) Lipiduria
(D) Pyuria
Q86. Which ketone body is detected by reagent strip testing?
(A) Acetoacetate
(B) All three equally
(C) Acetone
(D) β-hydroxybutyrate
Q87. Which urinary constituent causes a positive bilirubin reagent strip test but negative Ictotest?
(A) Conjugated bilirubin below sensitivity limit
(B) Ascorbic acid interference
(C) Urobilinogen
(D) Biliverdin
Q88. Which finding differentiates transudate from exudate in serous fluids?
(A) Cell type
(B) Protein and lactate dehydrogenase (LDH) levels
(C) Fluid volume
(D) Color and clarity
Q89. Xanthochromia in CSF indicates:
(A) Fungal infection
(B) Traumatic tap
(C) Bacterial meningitis
(D) Recent subarachnoid hemorrhage
Q90. The presence of oval fat bodies in urine is associated with:
(A) Hematuria
(B) Cystitis
(C) Acute glomerulonephritis
(D) Diabetes mellitus
Q91. A CSF WBC count showing primarily lymphocytes suggests:
(A) Bacterial meningitis
(B) Viral meningitis
(C) Parasitic infection
(D) Traumatic tap
Q92. Which urine pigment causes dark brown to black color upon standing due to oxidation?
(A) Bilirubin
(B) Melanin
(C) Hemoglobin
(D) Urobilinogen
Q93. Which finding indicates synovial fluid noninflammatory arthritis (e.g., osteoarthritis)?
(A) Low viscosity, high neutrophils
(B) Cloudy fluid with decreased glucose
(C) High viscosity, low WBC count
(D) Purulent appearance
Q94. Which crystals in acidic urine appear as yellow-brown spheres with concentric circles?
(A) Tyrosine
(B) Cystine
(C) Cholesterol
(D) Leucine

Q95. A positive CSF India ink test identifies which organism?
(A) Haemophilus influenzae
(B) Neisseria meningitidis
(C) Cryptococcus neoformans
(D) Listeria monocytogenes
Q96. Which urinary finding most strongly suggests glomerular bleeding rather than lower tract bleeding?
(A) Large numbers of squamous cells
(B) Epithelial cells and bacteria
(C) Dysmorphic red blood cells and RBC casts
(D) Uniform intact RBCs and mucus threads
Q97. A first-morning urine specimen is preferred for routine urinalysis because it:
(A) Is the most concentrated and stable
(B) Reflects average 24-hour excretion
(C) Minimizes bacterial contamination
(D) Is the most dilute
Q98. Tamm-Horsfall protein is secreted by which renal structure?
(A) Glomerulus
(B) Loop of Henle
(C) Distal convoluted tubule
(D) Renal tubular epithelial cells of the thick ascending limb
Q99. Which of the following is the most common cause of alkaline urine in a freshly voided sample?
(A) Vegetarian diet or postprandial alkalinity
(B) Starvation ketosis
(C) Renal tubular acidosis
(D) Dehydration
Q100. A urine specimen with positive nitrite and leukocyte esterase indicates:
(A) Bacterial urinary tract infection
(B) Contamination by vaginal flora
(C) Acute glomerulonephritis
(D) Sterile pyuria

Answer Key and Explanation (1-100)

Q1. Answer: B

Explanation: The D antigen is the most immunogenic of the Rh system because its exposure commonly elicits antibody formation following transfusion or pregnancy. Its high antigen density and strong membrane expression lead to robust immune responses. The other Rh antigens (C, c, E, e) are less immunogenic, producing weaker antibody reactions and lower rates of alloimmunization.

Q2. Answer: D

Explanation: Anti-D antibodies typically appear after exposure to Rh(D)-positive red cells, such as through pregnancy or transfusion. These IgG antibodies can cross the placenta and cause hemolytic disease of the fetus and newborn. Autoimmune or cold-reactive antibodies generally have broader thermal amplitude or different specificity, not limited to the D antigen.

Q3. Answer: B

Explanation: O negative blood lacks A, B, and Rh(D) antigens, minimizing risk of immune reaction in recipients of any type. It's the safest transfusion option in emergencies when crossmatching is unavailable. O positive could sensitize Rh-negative patients; AB types contain A and B antigens and are suitable only for plasma donation compatibility.

Q4. Answer: A

Explanation: IgG antibodies cross the placenta due to their small molecular size and Fc receptor-mediated transport. When maternal IgG reacts with fetal RBC antigens, it leads to hemolysis and anemia. IgM is too large to cross the placenta; IgA and IgD do not typically participate in hemolytic disease mechanisms.

Q5. Answer: B

Explanation: IgM antibodies are cold-reactive, showing peak agglutination at around 4°C. They are pentameric molecules, efficiently agglutinating red cells directly without antiglobulin reagents. IgG antibodies, in contrast, react best at 37°C and require antiglobulin testing. At higher temperatures, IgM loses binding efficiency and may dissociate.

Q6. Answer: B

Explanation: Proteolytic enzymes like ficin and papain destroy Duffy and MNS antigens but enhance Rh and Kidd antigen reactivity by exposing epitopes. Enzyme-treated cells thus strengthen reactions in Rh typing or antibody detection. Kell is enzyme-resistant and remains unaffected, so its reactivity pattern helps distinguish antibody specificities.

Q7. Answer: C

Explanation: A positive DAT detects antibodies or complement components bound directly to red cell surfaces inside the patient's body. It identifies autoimmune hemolytic anemia, hemolytic transfusion reactions, or HDN. Indirect antiglobulin tests instead detect antibodies circulating freely in serum. DAT thus differentiates in vivo sensitization from in vitro reactions.

Q8. Answer: B

Explanation: Polyspecific antiglobulin reagents contain antibodies against human IgG and complement component C3, allowing detection of either antibody- or complement-coated red cells. This dual reactivity enhances test sensitivity for autoimmune hemolytic and transfusion reactions. Reagents lacking these antibodies would yield false negatives in such conditions.

Q9. Answer: B

Explanation: The Duffy antigen (Fy^a/Fy^b) acts as a receptor for Plasmodium vivax. Individuals with the Fy(a-b-) phenotype, common in parts of Africa, are resistant to this malaria species. This selective advantage maintains the Duffy-null gene frequency. Kell, Kidd, and MNS have no known protective effects against malaria parasites.

Q10. Answer: C

Explanation: Delayed hemolytic transfusion reactions occur when an anamnestic IgG response targets transfused RBC antigens days after exposure. The IgG-coated cells undergo extravascular hemolysis. IgM antibodies usually cause immediate intravascular hemolysis. Cold autoantibodies cause benign agglutination without delayed onset.

Q11. Answer: B

Explanation: The saline replacement technique helps resolve rouleaux or protein-induced agglutination that mimics true antigen-antibody reactions, clarifying forward and reverse grouping discrepancies. DAT identifies cell-bound antibodies but not ABO mismatches. Secretor testing pertains to saliva antigen expression, not resolving rouleaux interference.

Q12. Answer: B

Explanation: Weak D testing identifies RBCs with reduced D antigen expression (partial or weak variants). Such cells may initially type as Rh-negative but react after incubation with antiglobulin reagent. Detecting these variants prevents sensitization and ensures correct Rh classification for donor units and recipients.

Q13. Answer: A

Explanation: EDTA chelates calcium, a necessary cofactor for complement activation. This prevents in vitro complement binding that could obscure antibody detection. Citrate and heparin are anticoagulants but do not specifically block complement. Sodium fluoride inhibits glycolysis, used mainly in glucose testing, not immunohematology.

Q14. Answer: C

Explanation: AB individuals possess both A and B antigens, so they lack corresponding antibodies. However, the person is Rh-negative, meaning no anti-D is naturally present but can be produced upon exposure. Type O individuals, not AB, have both anti-A and anti-B antibodies naturally formed due to environmental antigen exposure.

Q15. Answer: D

Explanation: The major crossmatch combines donor red cells with recipient serum to check for antibodies against donor antigens. It ensures transfused cells won't be destroyed by existing recipient antibodies. Minor crossmatch reverses this pairing but is obsolete due to screened donor units. Complement activity is not directly tested.

Q16. Answer: A

Explanation: Febrile non-hemolytic transfusion reactions result from leukocyte cytokines or recipient antibodies reacting to donor WBC antigens. Symptoms include fever and chills but no hemolysis. Allergic reactions involve urticaria or anaphylaxis; bacterial contamination causes rapid septic shock; acute hemolysis involves hemoglobinuria and renal injury.

Q17. Answer: B

Explanation: Rh immune globulin coats fetal Rh-positive cells in maternal circulation, promoting their rapid removal before maternal immune recognition. This prevents memory B-cell activation and anti-D production. It does not block antigen presentation directly nor stimulate IgG synthesis. Complement fixation isn't the protective mechanism.

Q18. Answer: D

Explanation: Enzyme treatments like papain degrade Duffy (Fy) antigens, weakening their reactivity. Rh and Kidd antigens are enhanced, while Kell remains stable. Recognizing enzyme-sensitive versus enzyme-resistant systems assists in antibody identification when mixed-field reactions occur during complex antibody workups.

Q19. Answer: A

Explanation: The IAT detects unbound IgG antibodies in patient serum by incubating with reagent RBCs, washing, and adding antiglobulin (Coombs) reagent. The polyspecific reagent contains anti-IgG ± anti-C3, bridging sensitized cells for visible agglutination. Lectins are used for ABO typing, not antibody screening.

Q20. Answer: C

Explanation: Inadequate washing leaves residual unbound globulins that neutralize antiglobulin reagent, preventing lattice formation and visible agglutination, thus yielding false negatives. Excess washing doesn't interfere; overcentrifugation may cause false positives. Aged serum affects antibody titers but not this specific step.

Q21. Answer: D

Explanation: Anti-I is usually a cold-reactive, naturally occurring IgM that does not cause hemolysis at body temperature, making it clinically insignificant. Anti-K, anti-Jka, and anti-D are IgG antibodies reacting at 37°C and can cause hemolytic transfusion reactions or HDN, hence considered clinically significant.

Q22. Answer: D

Explanation: Elution uses heat or acid to dissociate bound antibodies from red cell membranes for subsequent identification. Adsorption removes antibodies using target antigens, not elution. Gel filtration separates proteins by size but isn't for immunohematology. Enzyme-linked assays detect antibodies, not recover them.

Q23. Answer: D

Explanation: Kell antigens remain stable under enzyme treatment and provoke strong IgG responses capable of severe hemolytic disease and transfusion reactions. Their resistance to enzymatic degradation differentiates them from Duffy and MNS systems. Kell is expressed throughout life and clinically significant in both adults and neonates.

Q24. Answer: C

Explanation: Anti-A (and Anti-B) are potent naturally occurring IgM antibodies that activate complement, leading to acute intravascular hemolysis during ABO-incompatible transfusion. Anti-Lea and Anti-M are generally cold-reactive and mild; Anti-Jka may cause delayed, not immediate, hemolysis due to anamnestic IgG response.

Q25. Answer: B

Explanation: Kell-negative individuals may form anti-K antibodies after exposure to Kell-positive red cells, resulting in severe hemolytic transfusion reactions or HDN. The anti-K antibody is IgG, active at 37°C, and clinically significant. It's unrelated to autoimmunity, blood viscosity, or iron biochemistry.

Q26. Answer: C

Explanation: Adsorption studies remove autoantibodies using patient or donor red cells, allowing hidden alloantibodies to be detected in the adsorbed serum. This distinction guides safe transfusion selection. The direct antiglobulin test shows in-vivo coating but not antibody type, while saline replacement and forward grouping address rouleaux or ABO typing discrepancies, not antibody origin.

Q27. Answer: C

Explanation: Clinically important IgG antibodies react optimally at 37 °C and require the antiglobulin (AHG) phase for detection because they don't agglutinate directly. Cold or saline phases mainly show IgM activity. Complement fixation detects complement binding rather than specific RBC antibodies, so it's not part of routine antibody screens.

Q28. Answer: B

Explanation: LISS reduces the ionic concentration of the medium, decreasing repulsion between antibody and antigen sites, thus enhancing IgG uptake and shortening incubation time. It improves sensitivity of antibody screens. It does not remove existing IgG, destroy complement, or increase zeta potential-in fact, it lowers electrostatic forces for easier binding.

Q29. Answer: C

Explanation: The Kleihauer-Betke acid-elution test quantifies fetal RBCs in maternal blood, estimating hemorrhage volume to calculate required RhIG dose. The rosette screen is qualitative only. Indirect Coombs detects circulating antibodies, not fetal cell volume. Direct Coombs detects antibodies on neonatal cells, not maternal bleeding extent.

Q30. Answer: D

Explanation: Anti-Jka (Kidd system) antibodies often fade below detectable levels yet elicit rapid anamnestic IgG responses upon re-exposure, producing delayed hemolysis. Anti-K and Anti-E are significant but usually detected before transfusion. Anti-Lea is typically IgM, cold-reactive, and clinically mild, rarely causing delayed destruction of transfused cells.

Q31. Answer: A

Explanation: Duffy antigens demonstrate dosage-homozygous cells (Fy^aFy^a) react more strongly than heterozygous (Fy^aFy^b). Recognizing this pattern assists antibody identification. Lewis and P are not controlled by homozygosity in this way, and ABO antigens are codominant with equal expression, so dosage variability isn't a diagnostic feature for them.

Q32. Answer: A

Explanation: Packed RBCs are refrigerated at 1-6 °C to slow metabolism while preventing freezing. This preserves viability and reduces bacterial growth. Frozen RBCs require ≤ -65 °C, platelets are held at 20-24 °C with agitation, and plasma at ≤ -18 °C. Correct storage ensures antigen stability and patient safety during transfusion.

Q33. Answer: B

Explanation: Irradiation inactivates donor lymphocytes, preventing transfusion-associated graft-versus-host disease in immunocompromised or intrauterine transfusion recipients. It's unnecessary for routine anemias or iron deficiency. Autoimmune hemolysis requires antigen-matched, not irradiated, blood. Irradiation preserves RBC function but guarantees recipient safety in immune-suppressed conditions.

Q34. Answer: C

Explanation: Cryoprecipitate, derived from thawed FFP, contains concentrated fibrinogen, factor VIII, factor XIII, and von Willebrand factor. It's used for hypofibrinogenemia or DIC. Fresh frozen plasma has all coagulation factors but lower fibrinogen density. Platelet concentrates and albumin solutions serve different therapeutic roles, not fibrinogen replacement.

Q35. Answer: A

Explanation: Immediate cessation is essential in suspected acute hemolytic transfusion reaction to prevent further hemolysis. The IV line is kept open with saline, and both blood unit and samples are returned for investigation. Continuing the transfusion or delaying notification risks renal failure and severe hemolysis.

Q36. Answer: C

Explanation: Kell antigens remain unaffected by proteolytic enzymes such as papain or ficin, maintaining their antigenicity, whereas M, N, and Duffy antigens are degraded. This property aids in antibody identification when enzyme-treated panels alter reactivity patterns, helping differentiate overlapping antibody specificities during complex workups.

Q37. Answer: C

Explanation: An antibody screen uses reagent RBC panels to identify clinically significant unexpected antibodies. It's a key pretransfusion safeguard. The crossmatch pairs donor cells with recipient serum but follows screening. Direct Coombs assesses cell-bound IgG, not serum antibodies, and ABO typing alone misses non-ABO incompatibilities.

Q38. Answer: B

Explanation: Contaminated or rough glassware may promote nonspecific agglutination, leading to false-positive AHG results. Cold agglutinins can also yield spurious positives if testing occurs below 37 °C.

Overwashing removes excess serum and actually prevents false positives, while under-centrifugation may cause weak reactions rather than false positives.

Q39. Answer: B

Explanation: AB plasma lacks anti-A and anti-B antibodies, making it safe for recipients of all blood groups when only plasma is transfused. For red cells, O negative is universal donor, but plasma compatibility is reversed. Plasma from A or B donors contains respective antibodies that could react with recipient antigens.

Q40. Answer: B

Explanation: During storage, red cell metabolism continues, consuming glucose and lowering pH while 2,3-DPG levels fall, reducing oxygen delivery. Potassium leaks into plasma, increasing its concentration. These "storage lesions" are minimized by using additive solutions and limiting shelf life to preserve cell function.

Q41. Answer: A

Explanation: Anti-A and Anti-B are potent IgM antibodies that fix complement efficiently, causing rapid intravascular hemolysis during ABO incompatibility. Anti-K and Anti-D are IgG and cause mainly extravascular hemolysis. Anti-Fya rarely activates complement strongly. Recognizing complement-mediated hemolysis is vital for immediate reaction management.

Q42. Answer: C

Explanation: The antiglobulin (Coombs) test bridges IgG-coated RBCs, revealing sensitization invisible to the naked eye. It's used in antibody screening, crossmatching, and HDN investigation. It doesn't measure free antibody levels, hematocrit, or protein content-its purpose is detecting in-vivo or in-vitro cell sensitization.

Q43. Answer: B

Explanation: The D antigen defines Rh-positive status and is present in approximately 85 percent of most populations. C, c, and e are subsidiary Rh antigens that can coexist in various combinations, but D is the dominant determinant for Rh typing and alloimmunization risk.

Q44. Answer: B

Explanation: AS-1 (Adsol) solution adds adenine, dextrose, mannitol, and saline, supporting ATP production and membrane stability, extending RBC life to 42 days. CPD and CPDA-1 allow only 35 days; ACD-A is used for apheresis. Proper additive selection preserves cell viability and oxygen-delivery capacity during storage.

Q45. Answer: B

Explanation: Platelets are stored at room temperature (20-24 °C) with gentle agitation to preserve function and gas exchange. They expire after 5 days due to bacterial growth risk and metabolic decline. Refrigeration destroys platelet function, while extended storage requires pathogen-reduction and pH monitoring to maintain efficacy and safety.

Q46. Answer: C

Explanation: Factors V and VIII are the most labile coagulation factors. Rapid freezing of plasma within 8 hours preserves their activity. Factor V is particularly sensitive to temperature and storage time. Other factors (II, VII, X) remain stable longer, so delayed freezing would primarily impair Factor V levels and clinical effectiveness in replacement therapy.

Q47. Answer: B

Explanation: AB positive individuals possess A, B, and Rh(D) antigens and lack corresponding antibodies, so they can safely receive red cells from any group. However, their plasma can only be donated to AB recipients due to presence of anti-A/B antibodies in other types. Understanding reciprocal compatibility is crucial for emergency transfusion decisions.

Q48. Answer: D

Explanation: Therapeutic plasma exchange with fresh frozen plasma replaces deficient ADAMTS13 enzyme and removes inhibitors in TTP. Platelet transfusions are contraindicated because they worsen thrombosis. Cryoprecipitate and RBCs don't address the pathophysiology. Timely plasma therapy is life-saving by halting microvascular clot formation and organ damage.

Q49. Answer: B

Explanation: Blood bank refrigerators require daily temperature monitoring (1-6 °C for RBCs) with alarms and record charts to ensure regulatory compliance and product safety. pH, light, and humidity don't impact blood storage quality directly. Accurate temperature documentation verifies cold-chain integrity from collection to transfusion.

Q50. Answer: D

Explanation: Anti-K (Kell system) is the next most severe cause of hemolytic disease of the newborn after anti-D. It suppresses fetal erythropoiesis and causes severe anemia. Anti-Jkb and Anti-N may cause mild reactions; Anti-Lea is usually IgM and doesn't cross the placenta. Recognizing significant antibodies ensures early prophylaxis and monitoring.

Q51. Answer: C

Explanation: Washed RBCs remove nearly all plasma proteins and leukocytes, preventing recurrent or severe allergic transfusion reactions caused by plasma protein hypersensitivity. They're also used for IgA-deficient patients with anti-IgA antibodies. Washing doesn't treat iron deficiency or mild anemia and isn't needed for simple febrile reactions managed with leukoreduced units.

Q52. Answer: B

Explanation: Paroxysmal cold hemoglobinuria is caused by the biphasic Donath-Landsteiner antibody, a complement-binding IgG anti-P that sensitizes RBCs in the cold and causes lysis on warming. Anti-I and Anti-Lea are cold IgM antibodies but non-biphasic. Anti-D is clinically significant in HDN but unrelated to PCH mechanisms.

Q53. Answer: C

Explanation: A selected-cell panel includes reagent RBCs with known antigen profiles chosen to confirm or exclude multiple antibodies simultaneously. Enzyme panels alter antigen expression, aiding specificity confirmation but not primary identification. Saline crossmatch and forward typing are insufficient for detailed antibody characterization.

Q54. Answer: C

Explanation: Anti-A1 is a naturally occurring cold-reactive IgM found in a minority of A2 or A2B persons. It usually reacts below 30 °C and is rarely clinically significant. Its detection helps explain ABO reverse grouping discrepancies. Alloimmune IgG antibodies form after exposure; complement-dependent IgG describes warm autoantibodies, not Anti-A1.

Q55. Answer: A

Explanation: Autoadsorption removes autoantibodies using patient's own RBCs, but it's invalid after recent transfusion because donor cells would adsorb alloantibodies, masking their presence. It's appropriate for warm autoantibody cases using autologous cells only. Drug-induced or cold agglutinin cases require different diagnostic approaches, not adsorption-based methods.

Q56. Answer: C

Explanation: Albumin neutralizes negative surface charges between RBCs, reducing zeta potential andAllows IgG molecules to bridge cells more effectively. LISS accelerates antibody binding by ionic reduction; PEG removes water to concentrate antibodies; enzymes modify antigens. Albumin's mechanism uniquely enhances agglutination without altering antigens themselves.

Q57. Answer: B

Explanation: ABO-incompatible transfusions cause immediate intravascular hemolysis due to complement activation by naturally occurring IgM anti-A or anti-B. This leads to hemoglobinemia, hemoglobinuria, and potentially renal failure. Delayed hemolysis occurs days later from IgG alloantibodies, while febrile and urticarial reactions are much milder immune responses.

Q58. Answer: D

Explanation: The MNS antigen system resides on glycoproteins glycophorin A (M, N) and glycophorin B (S, s). These are sialoglycoproteins important for RBC membrane structure. Kell resides on a disulfide-linked protein, Duffy on a chemokine receptor, and Kidd on a urea transporter, each with different molecular sites.

Q59. Answer: A

Explanation: Frozen RBCs preserved in glycerol and stored at -65 °C or below remain viable for up to 10 years. Before transfusion, they must be thawed, deglycerolized, and used within 24 hours. This extended storage benefits rare donor units. Shorter durations apply to refrigerated or liquid-stored blood components.

Q60. Answer: C

Explanation: RhIG prevents maternal sensitization to Rh(D)-positive fetal RBCs by coating them for removal before antibody production. This prophylaxis prevents hemolytic disease of the newborn in future pregnancies. It has no effect on ABO incompatibility, GVHD, or febrile reactions, which involve distinct immune mechanisms and prophylactic measures.

Q61. Answer: C

Explanation: Rh-null individuals completely lack all Rh antigens (D, C, c, E, e). This rare condition causes hemolytic anemia and cell membrane abnormalities. Such patients can only receive Rh-null blood. Absence of a single antigen (e.g., D) results in partial Rh variants, not true Rh-null status.

Q62. Answer: C

Explanation: Clerical verification-matching patient name, ID number, and unit label-is the most critical step to prevent fatal errors. Most transfusion fatalities arise from clerical mistakes, not serologic mismatches. ABO typing, antibody screens, and crossmatches confirm compatibility but cannot prevent misidentification during specimen collection or transfusion.

Q63. Answer: C

Explanation: Cryoprecipitate provides concentrated factor VIII, fibrinogen, factor XIII, and vWF, ideal for treating hemophilia A or von Willebrand disease. FFP contains all coagulation factors but lower concentration; platelets don't correct clotting deficiencies. Whole blood is seldom used, as factor replacement and volume needs can be targeted more precisely with cryoprecipitate.

Q64. Answer: C

Explanation: Enzyme-treated RBCs expose Kidd antigens (Jka, Jkb), enhancing antibody reactivity. Enzymes destroy Duffy (Fya, Fyb) and MNS antigens, reducing their reactivity. Therefore, increased reaction after enzyme treatment indicates Kidd or Rh antibodies, aiding antibody differentiation in complex serologic patterns.

Q65. Answer: A

Explanation: Mixed-field agglutination occurs when two cell populations coexist-typically after transfusion with different group RBCs or marrow transplantation. One population agglutinates while the other remains unagglutinated, producing a mosaic pattern. Weak subgroups cause uniform weak reactions, and cold antibodies create broad nonspecific agglutination, not distinct populations.

Q66. Answer: B

Explanation: Performing elution on neonatal cells and identifying the eluted antibody confirms active hemolysis caused by maternal IgG. Passive antibody transfer yields weak DAT without clinical hemolysis. DAT alone shows coating but not specificity; the elution identifies the antibody responsible, guiding diagnosis and treatment of HDN severity.

Q67. Answer: D

Explanation: Newborns are Le(a-b-) because Lewis antigens are not intrinsic to RBCs but adsorbed from plasma later in life. Expression develops gradually as glycolipid production matures. Adult phenotypes Le(a+b-) or Le(a-b+) appear after several months. This explains Lewis system's lack of relevance in HDN due to absent fetal expression.

Q68. Answer: A

Explanation: Lewis antigens exist as soluble substances in secretor saliva. Mixing patient serum with secretor saliva neutralizes Lewis antibodies, confirming specificity. Enzymes enhance Lewis reactivity but don't neutralize; albumin affects zeta potential, and ficin treatment modifies cell antigens, not antibody removal. This principle helps antibody identification.

Q69. Answer: C

Explanation: Exchange transfusion in neonates requires O Rh-negative RBCs to avoid ABO/Rh incompatibility, irradiated to prevent GVHD, and CMV-negative to minimize infection risk. AB plasma alone doesn't correct anemia, platelets address thrombocytopenia, and random donor whole blood carries alloimmunization risks. Strict selection ensures neonatal safety.

Q70. Answer: A

Explanation: 2,3-DPG depletion reduces hemoglobin's ability to release oxygen to tissues, diminishing transfused RBC efficacy. ATP decline impairs membrane flexibility but less directly affects oxygen release. Elevated potassium and mild hemolysis are expected but reversible after transfusion. 2,3-DPG regeneration restores oxygen-carrying function post-transfusion.

Q71. Answer: A

Explanation: ADH, or vasopressin, acts on the distal tubules and collecting ducts to increase water permeability, allowing reabsorption and concentrating urine. Aldosterone mainly regulates sodium reabsorption and potassium excretion. ANP promotes natriuresis and diuresis, while renin initiates angiotensin formation for blood pressure control rather than direct water regulation.

Q72. Answer: D

Explanation: Specific gravity values above 1.030 often indicate interference from high molecular weight substances such as radiographic contrast media or glucose. Normal physiologic concentration rarely exceeds 1.030. Dilute urine shows low SG, and renal concentrating failure yields low fixed SG values. Confirm with reagent strip or osmolality testing.

Q73. Answer: C

Explanation: Highly alkaline urine can cause false-positive protein readings on the reagent strip by interfering with the color indicator reaction. The test relies on pH shift of a dye-buffer system sensitive to albumin. Glucose and ascorbic acid more commonly interfere with other analytes such as ketones or blood detection.

Q74. Answer: A

Explanation: When urine stands unpreserved at room temperature, bacteria multiply, converting nitrates to nitrites and increasing pH. This also produces ammonia odor and causes glucose and ketones to decrease due to bacterial metabolism and volatilization. WBCs and casts deteriorate over time, affecting microscopic examination accuracy.

Q75. Answer: B

Explanation: The glomerulus, a capillary tuft within Bowman's capsule, filters plasma under hydrostatic pressure, forming the initial ultrafiltrate. The loop of Henle and tubules modify filtrate composition through selective reabsorption and secretion. Collecting ducts concentrate urine under ADH influence but do not perform primary filtration.

Q76. Answer: C

Explanation: Myoglobin from muscle breakdown (rhabdomyolysis) produces a red, clear or hazy urine with a positive heme test and absence of RBCs. Hematuria shows intact RBCs microscopically. Menstrual contamination presents with epithelial cells and debris, while infection yields WBCs and bacteria, not isolated heme-positive pigment.

Q77. Answer: B

Explanation: The reagent strip glucose pad employs a two-step enzyme reaction: glucose oxidase converts glucose to gluconic acid and hydrogen peroxide; peroxidase then oxidizes a chromogen to yield color proportional to glucose concentration. The Clinitest (copper reduction) is nonspecific and reacts with any reducing substance, not exclusively glucose.

Q78. Answer: A

Explanation: RBC casts form within renal tubules when red cells are trapped in a Tamm-Horsfall protein matrix, indicating glomerular or tubular bleeding (e.g., glomerulonephritis). Lower tract bleeding lacks casts because casts form only in the renal tubules. Contamination or cystitis produces free RBCs, not casts.

Q79. Answer: C

Explanation: Cystine crystals are colorless, hexagonal plates characteristic of cystinuria, a congenital defect in amino acid transport. Tyrosine forms fine needles, leucine forms concentric spheres, and cholesterol forms notched plates. Recognition of cystine is crucial as it indicates a metabolic disorder predisposing to renal calculi formation.

Q80. Answer: A

Explanation: CSF glucose normally equals approximately two-thirds of plasma glucose due to selective transport across the blood-brain barrier. Low CSF glucose suggests bacterial infection, malignancy, or hypoglycemia. Values equal to plasma indicate hyperglycemia effect, while independent variation is physiologically implausible given barrier regulation.

Q81. Answer: D

Explanation: In chronic renal failure, tubules lose concentrating and diluting capacity, causing specific gravity to remain fixed near 1.010-the isosthenuric point matching plasma ultrafiltrate. Diabetes mellitus yields high SG from glucose; diabetes insipidus shows low SG due to water loss; dehydration temporarily increases SG, not fixes it.

Q82. Answer: C

Explanation: WBC casts reflect inflammation or infection within the renal parenchyma, characteristic of pyelonephritis or interstitial nephritis. They form when leukocytes are trapped in Tamm-Horsfall protein within renal tubules. Lower urinary tract infections produce free WBCs without casts; tubular necrosis yields granular or epithelial casts instead.

Q83. Answer: B

Explanation: Tamm-Horsfall protein (uromodulin), secreted by renal tubular epithelial cells, forms the protein matrix for all casts. It polymerizes under acidic, concentrated conditions. Albumin and hemoglobin may become incorporated but are not the structural basis. Recognizing Tamm-Horsfall origin differentiates renal from lower urinary tract elements.

Q84. Answer: B

Explanation: The Clinitest detects any reducing sugar (glucose, galactose, fructose) via copper reduction to cuprous oxide, producing color change. This broad sensitivity confirms presence of sugars missed by glucose oxidase-specific strips. Ictotest detects bilirubin; Acetest detects ketones. Thus, Clinitest helps diagnose inborn errors like galactosemia.

Q85. Answer: B

Explanation: Phosphates precipitate in alkaline urine, giving a cloudy or milky appearance. They dissolve upon acidification with acetic acid, confirming phosphaturia. Pyuria (WBCs) and chyluria (lymphatic leakage) persist after acid addition; lipiduria demonstrates fat globules under microscopy, unaffected by pH change.

Q86. Answer: A

Explanation: The reagent strip nitroprusside reaction detects acetoacetate most sensitively and acetone weakly, but not β-hydroxybutyrate. In diabetic ketoacidosis, β-hydroxybutyrate predominates; thus, strips may underestimate severity. Confirmatory blood testing for β-hydroxybutyrate provides more accurate assessment of metabolic ketoacid status in critical care settings.

Q87. Answer: A

Explanation: The Ictotest is more sensitive; a negative Ictotest following a positive strip suggests trace conjugated bilirubin below confirmatory detection threshold. Urobilinogen reacts on a different pad; biliverdin doesn't react; ascorbic acid causes false negatives, not this discrepancy. Trace conjugated bilirubin still reflects early hepatic dysfunction.

Q88. Answer: B

Explanation: Transudates result from systemic factors like pressure or oncotic imbalance and show low protein and LDH (<0.5 of serum). Exudates, due to inflammation, have high protein and LDH. Light's criteria use these ratios for classification. Color or cell count helps but lacks diagnostic precision compared to biochemical indices.

Q89. Answer: D

Explanation: Xanthochromia, a yellow discoloration of supernatant CSF, arises from bilirubin breakdown after intracranial bleeding, confirming true subarachnoid hemorrhage. Traumatic taps show clearing in successive tubes without xanthochromia. Infections cause turbidity, not yellow pigment. Xanthochromia persists hours after bleeding, aiding retrospective hemorrhage confirmation.

Q90. Answer: D

Explanation: Oval fat bodies-lipid-laden renal tubular cells-appear in lipiduria of nephrotic syndrome, often secondary to diabetes mellitus. They show Maltese crosses under polarized light. Glomerulonephritis yields RBC casts, cystitis produces WBCs, and hematuria shows free RBCs. Fat bodies signify significant proteinuria and lipid metabolism disturbance in renal disease.

Q91. Answer: B

Explanation: Viral meningitis typically produces lymphocytic predominance in CSF with moderate WBC elevation, normal or slightly elevated protein, and normal glucose. Bacterial meningitis yields neutrophilic predominance and very high protein with low glucose. Parasitic infections show eosinophils; traumatic taps mainly introduce peripheral blood elements.

Q92. Answer: B

Explanation: Melanin precursors in urine oxidize to dark brown or black on standing, suggesting metastatic melanoma. Hemoglobin darkens red, bilirubin gives yellow foam, and urobilinogen oxidizes to urobilin with lighter brown hue. Identifying melaninuria alerts clinicians to malignant melanoma metastasis.

Q93. Answer: C

Explanation: Noninflammatory arthritis yields clear, viscous synovial fluid with low WBC count (<2000/μL) and normal glucose. Inflammatory or infectious forms decrease viscosity and increase neutrophil content. Purulence implies infection. High viscosity reflects intact hyaluronic acid polymerization, typical in degenerative, noninflammatory conditions.

Q94. Answer: D

Explanation: Leucine crystals are yellow-brown concentric spheres with radial striations, seen in severe liver disease. Tyrosine appears as fine colorless needles, cystine as colorless hexagons, and cholesterol as notched plates. These abnormal crystals indicate hepatic dysfunction and protein metabolism abnormalities.

Q95. Answer: C

Explanation: The India ink preparation reveals encapsulated Cryptococcus neoformans by demonstrating a clear halo around yeast cells. This fungus commonly infects immunocompromised patients causing meningitis. Other bacterial pathogens are visualized via Gram stain. India ink's negative contrast microscopy highlights the thick polysaccharide capsule unique to Cryptococcus.

Q96. Answer: C

Explanation: Dysmorphic RBCs and RBC casts indicate glomerular origin because red cells become deformed while passing through damaged glomerular membranes. RBC casts form within renal tubules, confirming intrarenal bleeding. Uniform RBCs suggest lower tract bleeding, and epithelial cells or squamous contamination indicate nonrenal sources. Recognizing dysmorphic RBC morphology differentiates nephritic from postrenal hematuria.

Q97. Answer: A

Explanation: First-morning urine is concentrated due to overnight water reabsorption, allowing maximal detection of abnormal constituents such as protein or cells. It's less affected by recent fluid intake. Though relatively sterile, its key advantage is concentration and stability for both chemical and microscopic testing. Random samples may miss early pathologic changes.

Q98. Answer: D

Explanation: Tamm-Horsfall protein (uromodulin) is produced by epithelial cells of the thick ascending limb and distal convoluted tubule. It forms the matrix of casts and serves protective and anti-bacterial roles in the urinary tract. It is absent from glomerular filtrate, distinguishing tubular secretion products from plasma-derived proteins.

Q99. Answer: A

Explanation: Alkaline urine most often results from a vegetarian diet rich in fruits and vegetables or after meals when bicarbonate excretion increases (postprandial alkalinity). Renal tubular acidosis usually produces variable pH, while starvation and dehydration create acidic urine due to ketone or acid accumulation. Fresh sample pH reflects metabolic and dietary influence.

Q100. Answer: A

Explanation: Positive nitrite (nitrate reduction by bacteria) and leukocyte esterase (WBC enzyme) strongly suggest urinary tract infection by nitrate-reducing organisms such as E. coli. Glomerulonephritis and sterile pyuria lack bacterial nitrate conversion. Contamination may yield false positives but rarely shows both tests positive together, making combined reactivity diagnostic for bacterial UTI.

Question (101-200)

Q101. Which urinary cast type indicates chronic renal failure and severe tubular stasis?

(A) Waxy
(B) Hyaline
(C) Cellular
(D) Granular

Q103. Which finding is most consistent with nephrotic syndrome?

(A) Epithelial casts and renal failure
(B) Fatty casts and oval fat bodies
(C) WBC casts and pyuria
(D) RBC casts and hematuria

Q104. Which of the following best describes isosthenuria?

(A) Dilute urine less than 1.005
(B) Constant specific gravity around 1.010
(C) Increased osmolality due to dehydration
(D) Concentrated urine greater than 1.030

Q107. Amorphous phosphates are typically found in which type of urine?

(A) Acidic
(B) Neutral
(C) Any pH
(D) Alkaline

Q109. Which urinary condition yields colorless, dilute urine with low specific gravity?

(A) Hematuria
(B) Dehydration
(C) Diabetes insipidus
(D) Acute glomerulonephritis

Q110. WBC casts in urine are most characteristic of:

(A) Cystitis
(B) Prostatitis
(C) Pyelonephritis
(D) Urethritis

Q111. The nitroprusside reaction detects which compound?

(A) Glucose
(B) Protein
(C) Bilirubin
(D) Ketones

Q112. In CSF analysis, a high protein with normal glucose and lymphocytes indicates:

(A) Viral meningitis
(B) Fungal infection
(C) Bacterial meningitis
(D) Subarachnoid hemorrhage

Q113. Which urine preservative best maintains cellular elements for delayed microscopy?

(A) Formalin
(B) Refrigeration
(C) Toluene
(D) Hydrochloric acid

Q114. Leucine and tyrosine crystals in acidic urine indicate:

(A) Diabetes mellitus
(B) Dehydration
(C) Liver disease
(D) Starvation ketosis

Q115. Which CSF test helps distinguish subarachnoid hemorrhage from a traumatic tap?
(A) Elevated glucose concentration
(B) Gram stain
(C) Xanthochromia after centrifugation
(D) Clot formation after standing

Q116. Which finding supports tubular proteinuria?
(A) Presence of albumin only
(B) Negative protein electrophoresis
(C) Presence of low-molecular-weight proteins (β2-microglobulin)
(D) Positive sulfosalicylic acid test only

Q117. Which body fluid normally contains the highest hyaluronic acid concentration?
(A) Synovial fluid
(B) Amniotic fluid
(C) CSF
(D) Pleural fluid

Q118. Which test result combination indicates diabetes mellitus rather than starvation ketosis?
(A) Negative ketones, positive protein
(B) Positive glucose and ketones
(C) Negative glucose, positive ketones
(D) Positive bilirubin, negative glucose

Q119. Which finding differentiates exudate from transudate pleural fluid?
(A) Glucose value
(B) Appearance only
(C) Protein and LDH ratios to serum
(D) Cell count alone

Q120. In CSF analysis, elevated protein and RBCs without xanthochromia suggest:
(A) Traumatic tap
(B) Bacterial meningitis
(C) Viral meningitis
(D) Subarachnoid hemorrhage

Q121. Which enzyme is most specific for acute myocardial infarction (AMI) diagnosis?
(A) Creatine kinase-MB (CK-MB)
(B) Lactate dehydrogenase (LDH)
(C) Troponin I
(D) Aspartate aminotransferase (AST)

Q122. Indirect bilirubin represents bilirubin that is:
(A) Conjugated with glucuronic acid
(B) Bound to albumin and water-insoluble
(C) Excreted in bile
(D) Present in urine

Q123. The anion gap is calculated using which equation?
(A) $(Na^+ - Cl^-) / K^+$
(B) $(Na^+ + K^+) - (Cl^- + HCO_3^-)$
(C) $(Na^+ + Cl^-) - HCO_3^-$

(D) $(Na^+ + Ca^{2+}) - (K^+ + Cl^-)$

Q125. Which of the following conditions causes respiratory alkalosis?

(A) Chronic obstructive pulmonary disease

(B) Hypoventilation

(C) Salicylate overdose in late stages

(D) Anxiety-induced hyperventilation

Q126. Which electrolyte imbalance most commonly produces cardiac arrhythmias?

(A) Hyperchloremia

(B) Hypocalcemia

(C) Hyperkalemia

(D) Hyponatremia

Q127. Hemoglobin A1c reflects mean plasma glucose concentration over approximately:

(A) 1 week

(B) 2-3 months

(C) 1 month

(D) 6 months

Q128. Which enzyme catalyzes the conversion of creatine phosphate to creatine, releasing energy?

(A) CK (Creatine kinase)

(B) ALT

(C) LDH

(D) AST

Q130. Which test best assesses renal glomerular filtration rate (GFR)?

(A) Serum creatinine

(B) Creatinine clearance

(C) Blood ammonia

(D) Serum urea nitrogen

Q131. The primary function of albumin in plasma is:

(A) Oxygen binding

(B) Maintenance of oncotic pressure and transport

(C) Blood clotting

(D) Immune defense

Q132. Which lipoprotein transports cholesterol from tissues to the liver for excretion?

(A) Chylomicrons

(B) VLDL

(C) LDL

(D) HDL

Q133. Which enzyme system is responsible for detoxifying hydrogen peroxide in cells?

(A) Oxidase

(B) Transaminase

(C) Catalase

(D) Dehydrogenase

Q135. Which electrolyte maintains the resting membrane potential and intracellular fluid balance?

(A) Potassium

(B) Sodium

(C) Calcium

(D) Chloride

Q137. Thyroid-stimulating hormone (TSH) secretion is regulated by:

(A) Glucose concentration

(B) ACTH from the pituitary
(C) Feedback inhibition by T_3 and T_4
(D) Cortisol levels
Q138. Which enzyme shows highest elevation in acute pancreatitis?
(A) ALT
(B) Amylase
(C) Lipase
(D) LDH
Q140. Which lipid measurement correlates most strongly with atherosclerotic risk?
(A) VLDL cholesterol
(B) LDL cholesterol
(C) HDL cholesterol
(D) Triglycerides
Q141. In metabolic alkalosis, laboratory findings include:
(A) Decreased pH, normal bicarbonate
(B) Increased pH and bicarbonate
(C) Increased pH, decreased bicarbonate
(D) Decreased pH and bicarbonate
Q142. Which hormone promotes renal reabsorption of sodium and excretion of potassium?
(A) Renin
(B) Aldosterone
(C) ADH
(D) Cortisol
Q143. Gamma-glutamyl transferase (GGT) is particularly useful for detecting:
(A) Acute viral hepatitis
(B) Alcoholic liver disease
(C) Skeletal muscle injury
(D) Myocardial infarction
Q144. Which laboratory test best evaluates long-term glucose control in diabetic patients?
(A) Serum fructosamine
(B) Fasting plasma glucose
(C) HbA1c
(D) Oral glucose tolerance test
Q146. Which enzyme elevation is most characteristic of hepatocellular injury?
(A) Creatine kinase (CK)
(B) Lipase
(C) Alanine aminotransferase (ALT)
(D) Alkaline phosphatase (ALP)
Q147. Which thyroid profile suggests primary hypothyroidism?
(A) High TSH, low T_4
(B) High TSH, high T_4
(C) Low TSH, low T_4
(D) Low TSH, high T_4
Q148. The BUN:creatinine ratio is most useful for differentiating:
(A) Protein from carbohydrate metabolism
(B) Prerenal from intrinsic renal azotemia
(C) Hepatic from renal disease
(D) Acute vs. chronic renal failure

Q149. Which test best assesses acid-base status in blood?
(A) Arterial blood gas (ABG) analysis
(B) Urine pH
(C) Serum bicarbonate alone
(D) Serum CO_2
Q150. In iron deficiency anemia, which pattern is expected?
(A) High serum iron, low TIBC, high ferritin
(B) High serum iron, high TIBC
(C) Low serum iron, high TIBC, low ferritin
(D) Low serum iron, high ferritin
Q151. Hyperammonemia is most indicative of:
(A) Diabetes mellitus
(B) Renal failure
(C) Pancreatitis
(D) Hepatic dysfunction
Q152. Which enzyme is most useful in diagnosing prostate carcinoma?
(A) ALT
(B) GGT
(C) Alkaline phosphatase (ALP)
(D) Acid phosphatase (ACP)
Q153. Which blood component is primarily responsible for buffering metabolic acids?
(A) Hemoglobin
(B) Plasma proteins
(C) Phosphate
(D) Bicarbonate
Q154. Which glucose tolerance curve indicates diabetes mellitus?
(A) Fasting <100 mg/dL, 2-hr <140 mg/dL
(B) Fasting 110 mg/dL, 2-hr 100 mg/dL
(C) Fasting 126 mg/dL or greater, 2-hr ≥200 mg/dL
(D) Fasting 70 mg/dL, 2-hr 120 mg/dL
Q156. Glycosylated hemoglobin (HbA1c) increases in proportion to:
(A) Insulin secretion
(B) Serum fructosamine
(C) RBC turnover rate
(D) Average plasma glucose concentration
Q157. Hemolysis interferes most with measurement of:
(A) Calcium and phosphate
(B) Glucose and creatinine
(C) Sodium and chloride
(D) Potassium and LDH
Q158. Which enzyme is elevated earliest after myocardial infarction?
(A) CK-MB
(B) AST
(C) LDH
(D) Troponin I
Q159. Lactate accumulation in blood indicates:
(A) Enhanced aerobic metabolism
(B) Tissue hypoxia and anaerobic metabolism

(C) Alkalosis
(D) Reduced carbohydrate intake

Q161. Hypernatremia most commonly results from:
(A) Addison's disease
(B) Excessive sodium intake
(C) Syndrome of inappropriate ADH
(D) Water loss exceeding sodium loss

Q162. Which condition elevates both AST and ALT but normal ALP?
(A) Bone disease
(B) Hepatocellular injury
(C) Biliary obstruction
(D) Alcoholic cirrhosis with cholestasis

Q163. Hypoglycemia in adults is most frequently caused by:
(A) Adrenal insufficiency
(B) Thyrotoxicosis
(C) Insulinoma or excess insulin administration
(D) Liver cirrhosis

Q164. Which lipoprotein fraction is rich in triglycerides and appears after a fatty meal?
(A) VLDL
(B) LDL
(C) HDL
(D) Chylomicrons

Q166. Uric acid crystals in urine are associated with:
(A) Gout or high purine turnover
(B) Renal tubular acidosis
(C) Diabetes mellitus
(D) Bacterial infection

Q168. Which test detects creatinine in urine by colorimetric reaction with picric acid in alkaline solution?
(A) Van den Bergh test
(B) Jaffe reaction
(C) Biuret method
(D) Folin-Wu method

Q169. High ALP and GGT with normal AST/ALT suggests:
(A) Muscle disease
(B) Bone fracture
(C) Acute hepatitis
(D) Obstructive jaundice or cholestasis

Q170. Hypercalcemia due to parathyroid adenoma is characterized by:
(A) Low PTH and low phosphate
(B) High PTH and high phosphate
(C) High PTH and low phosphate
(D) Low PTH and high phosphate

Q171. Which enzyme is most specific for liver disease due to alcohol abuse?
(A) GGT
(B) ALT
(C) ALP
(D) AST

Q173. Hyperchloremic metabolic acidosis typically results from:
(A) Lactic acidosis
(B) Diarrhea or renal tubular acidosis
(C) Salicylate poisoning
(D) Diabetic ketoacidosis
Q174. In Cushing's syndrome, plasma cortisol levels are:
(A) Increased due to adrenal hyperfunction
(B) Normal with increased aldosterone
(C) Decreased from pituitary suppression
(D) Decreased with increased ACTH
Q176. The most sensitive test for early diabetic nephropathy is:
(A) Urine dipstick for protein
(B) Serum creatinine
(C) Microalbuminuria detection
(D) Creatinine clearance
Q178. Which plasma protein increases during inflammation as an acute-phase reactant?
(A) Transferrin
(B) Albumin
(C) Prealbumin
(D) C-reactive protein (CRP)
Q179. Serum osmolality can be roughly estimated by:
(A) $(2 \times Na^+) + (Glucose/18) + (BUN/2.8)$
(B) $(Na^+ + K^+ + Cl^-)/3$
(C) $(Na^+ \times Cl^-)/BUN$
(D) $(2 \times K^+) + Glucose$
Q180. Which test best evaluates adrenal medulla function?
(A) Plasma cortisol
(B) Aldosterone levels
(C) Serum renin activity
(D) Urinary catecholamines or metanephrines
Q181. Prolonged fasting primarily elevates which blood component?
(A) Insulin
(B) Glucose
(C) Free fatty acids and ketones
(D) Amino acids
Q182. Which vitamin deficiency causes megaloblastic anemia and elevated homocysteine and methylmalonic acid?
(A) Vitamin B_6
(B) Niacin
(C) Vitamin B_{12}
(D) Folic acid
Q183. Respiratory alkalosis may result from:
(A) COPD
(B) Metabolic acidosis
(C) Hypoventilation
(D) Hyperventilation due to anxiety or fever
Q184. Which condition causes both increased serum calcium and PTH?
(A) Malignancy

(B) Primary hyperparathyroidism
(C) Chronic renal failure
(D) Vitamin D deficiency
Q185. Which enzyme catalyzes the reversible conversion of lactate to pyruvate?
(A) ALT
(B) CK
(C) LDH
(D) AST
Q186. Which electrolyte imbalance is characteristic of Addison's disease?
(A) Hyponatremia and hyperkalemia
(B) Hypernatremia and hyperkalemia
(C) Hyponatremia and hypokalemia
(D) Hypernatremia and hypokalemia
Q187. Which analyte increases significantly in obstructive jaundice but not hemolytic anemia?
(A) LDH
(B) Unconjugated bilirubin
(C) Conjugated bilirubin
(D) Urobilinogen
Q188. Troponin T and I levels are primarily used to:
(A) Detect myocardial infarction
(B) Diagnose hepatic failure
(C) Evaluate renal function
(D) Confirm muscle dystrophy
Q189. Which enzyme increases in both liver and bone disorders?
(A) LDH
(B) ALP
(C) ALT
(D) GGT
Q192. Which protein fraction increases most during chronic inflammation?
(A) β-globulins
(B) γ-globulins
(C) Albumin
(D) α_1-globulins
Q193. In acute pancreatitis, which pair of enzymes shows the most significant increase?
(A) ALT and AST
(B) CK and LDH
(C) Amylase and Lipase
(D) GGT and ALP
Q194. Which serum enzyme is the most useful indicator of cholestasis?
(A) ALT
(B) ALP
(C) CK-MB
(D) AST
Q195. Low serum phosphorus with high calcium is characteristic of:
(A) Hypoparathyroidism
(B) Renal failure
(C) Vitamin D intoxication
(D) Primary hyperparathyroidism

Q196. Which test confirms the diagnosis of phenylketonuria (PKU)?

(A) Guthrie bacterial inhibition test

(B) Benedict's test

(C) Clinitest

(D) Rothera's test

Q197. Hypochloremic metabolic alkalosis is most often due to:

(A) Salicylate poisoning

(B) Ketoacidosis

(C) Vomiting or gastric suction

(D) Diarrhea

Q199. Which glucose method is most specific for measuring plasma glucose?

(A) Glucose oxidase

(B) Clinitest

(C) Copper reduction

(D) Benedict's method

Q200. Which hormone increases blood glucose by stimulating glycogenolysis and gluconeogenesis?

(A) Glucagon

(B) Aldosterone

(C) Insulin

(D) Calcitonin

Answer Key and Explanation (101-200)

Q101. Answer: A

Explanation: Waxy casts form from degenerated granular casts in prolonged stasis, reflecting chronic renal failure. They appear highly refractile with blunt ends and notched borders. Hyaline casts are nonspecific; granular casts show earlier degeneration; cellular casts reflect acute injury. Waxy forms signify the final stage of cast evolution and chronic tubular damage.

Q103. Answer: B

Explanation: Nephrotic syndrome causes heavy proteinuria leading to lipiduria; lipids are reabsorbed by renal cells forming oval fat bodies and fatty casts. These appear as Maltese crosses under polarized light. RBC casts indicate nephritic processes, WBC casts infection, and epithelial casts tubular injury. Lipiduria distinguishes nephrotic pathology from inflammatory renal conditions.

Q104. Answer: B

Explanation: Isosthenuria denotes fixed urine specific gravity (~1.010), identical to plasma ultrafiltrate, indicating renal tubules have lost concentrating and diluting ability. It's typical of chronic renal failure. Very low or high SG values show preserved tubular function. Monitoring SG trends helps assess renal concentrating capacity in progressive kidney disease.

Q107. Answer: D

Explanation: Amorphous phosphates precipitate in alkaline urine, appearing as fine, colorless granules that dissolve with acetic acid. Amorphous urates occur in acidic urine and dissolve with heat. Distinguishing these helps avoid misidentifying nonpathologic precipitates as pathological crystals. Urine pH guides crystal type interpretation in microscopy.

Q109. Answer: C

Explanation: Diabetes insipidus results from ADH deficiency or resistance, causing excessive water loss, dilute urine, and low SG (<1.005). Dehydration increases concentration; glomerulonephritis often yields protein and RBCs; hematuria adds color but not dilution. Persistent hypotonic urine despite dehydration is diagnostic of diabetes insipidus.

Q110. Answer: C

Explanation: WBC casts indicate infection within the renal parenchyma, typical of pyelonephritis. In cystitis or urethritis, WBCs appear free, not in casts, since these infections affect lower urinary tract sites. Casts form only within renal tubules; thus, WBC casts confirm upper tract involvement requiring systemic antibiotic therapy.

Q111. Answer: D

Explanation: The nitroprusside reaction detects acetoacetic acid (a ketone body) by color formation when nitroprusside reacts with acetoacetate and alkaline buffer. This is the principle of the Acetest and urine dipstick ketone pad. Glucose uses glucose oxidase; bilirubin uses diazo reaction; protein relies on pH indicators. Nitroprusside ensures ketone specificity.

Q112. Answer: A

Explanation: Viral meningitis typically elevates CSF protein moderately while glucose remains normal and lymphocytes predominate. Bacterial infections show very high protein with low glucose and neutrophils. Subarachnoid hemorrhage adds RBCs; fungal infections lower glucose variably. The mild, lymphocytic, normal-glucose pattern distinguishes viral inflammation from bacterial or hemorrhagic processes.

Q113. Answer: B

Explanation: Refrigeration slows bacterial growth and cellular degradation, preserving casts and cells up to 24 hours. Chemical preservatives like formalin alter chemical tests, while acids or toluene distort morphology. Thus, refrigeration is preferred for delayed examination when prompt analysis isn't possible, ensuring accuracy across all test categories.

Q114. Answer: C

Explanation: Leucine and tyrosine crystals appear in severe hepatic impairment due to disturbed amino acid metabolism. Tyrosine forms fine needles; leucine forms concentric spheres. These abnormal crystals signify advanced liver failure. Diabetes and ketosis produce ketone bodies; dehydration concentrates solutes but not amino acid crystals. Identification aids hepatic disease detection.

Q115. Answer: C

Explanation: Xanthochromia-yellow supernatant due to bilirubin-appears after subarachnoid hemorrhage, confirming true bleeding. In traumatic tap, successive tubes show decreasing blood without xanthochromia. CSF clot formation occurs with increased fibrin, not bleeding type. Measuring xanthochromia provides retrospective confirmation even hours after hemorrhage onset.

Q116. Answer: C

Explanation: Tubular proteinuria results from defective reabsorption of low-molecular-weight proteins (β2-microglobulin, retinol-binding protein). It differs from glomerular proteinuria (albumin) and overflow types (hemoglobin, myoglobin). Detection of these specific proteins indicates proximal tubular dysfunction due to drugs, toxins, or ischemia. Confirm by electrophoresis or immunoassay.

Q117. Answer: A

Explanation: Synovial fluid's viscosity arises from high hyaluronic acid content produced by synoviocytes, serving as a lubricant for joint movement. Its degradation decreases viscosity in inflammatory arthritis. CSF and pleural fluids contain minimal hyaluronate, while amniotic fluid has other mucopolysaccharides. Measuring viscosity aids arthritis classification.

Q118. Answer: B

Explanation: Diabetes mellitus produces both hyperglycemia and ketoacidosis, leading to positive glucose and ketone results. Starvation ketosis shows ketones only due to fat metabolism with normal glucose. Bilirubin and protein relate to hepatic or renal conditions, not carbohydrate metabolism. Combined glucose and ketone positivity is diagnostic for diabetic ketoacidosis.

Q119. Answer: C

Explanation: Exudates have high protein and LDH relative to serum (>0.5 and >0.6 respectively) due to increased vascular permeability from inflammation or malignancy. Transudates result from systemic factors like heart failure and show low ratios. Cell counts vary with cause, and glucose helps in infection diagnosis but not classification.

Q120. Answer: A

Explanation: A traumatic tap introduces peripheral blood during puncture, causing elevated RBCs and protein but no xanthochromia since RBCs haven't degraded to bilirubin. Subarachnoid hemorrhage develops xanthochromia after several hours. Bacterial meningitis raises WBCs and protein with low glucose, not RBCs. Sequential tube clearing confirms traumatic origin.

Q121. Answer: C

Explanation: Cardiac troponin I is the most specific and sensitive biomarker for AMI. It appears within 4-6 hours of myocardial injury and remains elevated for up to 7-10 days. CK-MB rises earlier but lacks complete specificity; AST and LDH elevations occur in many tissues. Troponin I directly reflects myocardial cell damage, confirming cardiac necrosis.

Q122. Answer: B

Explanation: Indirect (unconjugated) bilirubin is produced from hemoglobin catabolism, transported bound to albumin, and is water-insoluble. It becomes conjugated in the liver by glucuronyl transferase, forming direct bilirubin that is water-soluble and excreted in bile. Indirect bilirubin cannot appear in urine due to albumin binding and insolubility.

Q123. Answer: B

Explanation: Anion gap = $(Na^+ + K^+) - (Cl^- + HCO_3^-)$, though K^+ is sometimes omitted due to low concentration. It reflects unmeasured anions (lactate, phosphates, sulfates) and aids metabolic acidosis diagnosis. Elevated anion gap suggests acid accumulation, while normal gap indicates bicarbonate loss. Accurate electrolyte values are crucial for interpretation.

Q125. Answer: D

Explanation: Hyperventilation during anxiety decreases CO_2 levels, reducing carbonic acid and elevating blood pH-classic respiratory alkalosis. COPD and hypoventilation cause respiratory acidosis. Late salicylate toxicity shifts to metabolic acidosis after initial respiratory alkalosis. Identifying respiratory vs. metabolic sources requires arterial blood gas analysis correlating pH, pCO_2, and HCO_3^-.

Q126. Answer: C

Explanation: Hyperkalemia reduces myocardial excitability threshold, causing peaked T-waves, widened QRS, and potential cardiac arrest. Potassium profoundly influences membrane potentials. Hyponatremia and chloride disturbances mainly affect CNS and acid-base balance; hypocalcemia causes neuromuscular irritability, not arrhythmia. Continuous ECG monitoring is critical in suspected hyperkalemia.

Q127. Answer: B

Explanation: Hemoglobin A1c measures glycation of hemoglobin over the 120-day lifespan of red cells, reflecting average glucose levels over 2-3 months. It is unaffected by daily fluctuations and serves as a long-term glycemic control index. Shorter durations (e.g., fructosamine) assess recent glycemia, while HbA1c provides a chronic trend indicator.

Q128. Answer: A

Explanation: Creatine kinase (CK) transfers phosphate from creatine phosphate to ADP, regenerating ATP in muscle tissue. CK isoenzymes (CK-MM, CK-MB, CK-BB) are tissue-specific, aiding diagnosis of myocardial or muscular injury. ALT and AST are transaminases for amino acid metabolism; LDH catalyzes lactate-pyruvate interconversion, not ATP regeneration.

Q130. Answer: B

Explanation: Creatinine clearance measures the volume of plasma cleared of creatinine per minute, directly estimating GFR. It requires timed urine collection and serum creatinine measurement. Serum creatinine alone reflects renal function but not filtration rate precisely. Urea is influenced by diet and hydration; ammonia assesses hepatic detoxification, not filtration.

Q131. Answer: B

Explanation: Albumin maintains plasma oncotic pressure, preventing fluid leakage from capillaries, and serves as a carrier for bilirubin, hormones, drugs, and fatty acids. It is not involved in coagulation or oxygen transport. Low albumin levels lead to edema and altered drug binding. It's synthesized by the liver and reduced in hepatic failure.

Q132. Answer: D

Explanation: High-density lipoprotein (HDL) mediates reverse cholesterol transport-carrying cholesterol from peripheral tissues to the liver for conversion to bile acids. LDL delivers cholesterol to tissues, promoting atherogenesis. VLDL carries triglycerides, and chylomicrons transport dietary lipids. HDL's cardioprotective role makes it a key marker for cardiovascular risk assessment.

Q133. Answer: C

Explanation: Catalase, present in peroxisomes, decomposes hydrogen peroxide into water and oxygen, preventing oxidative damage. It acts rapidly and protects cellular structures. Oxidases generate hydrogen peroxide during metabolism; transaminases and dehydrogenases are involved in amino acid and carbohydrate metabolism, respectively. Catalase deficiency increases oxidative stress risk.

Q135. Answer: A

Explanation: Potassium is the major intracellular cation responsible for maintaining resting membrane potential and neuromuscular excitability. The Na^+/K^+ ATPase pump preserves its intracellular predominance. Sodium regulates extracellular osmolarity, calcium supports bone and clotting functions, and chloride balances cationic charges. Potassium imbalance immediately affects cardiac and nerve function.

Q137. Answer: C
Explanation: TSH release from the anterior pituitary is regulated by negative feedback from circulating thyroxine (T_4) and triiodothyronine (T_3). When thyroid hormone levels rise, TSH secretion decreases. ACTH regulates cortisol, not thyroid hormones. Glucose levels affect insulin, not TSH. This axis maintains euthyroid metabolic balance.

Q138. Answer: C
Explanation: Serum lipase is the most specific marker for acute pancreatitis and remains elevated longer than amylase. Amylase also rises but lacks specificity due to salivary isoforms. ALT and LDH are hepatic and general tissue enzymes. Elevated lipase confirms pancreatic origin of abdominal pain, guiding targeted management.

Q140. Answer: B
Explanation: LDL cholesterol carries the majority of plasma cholesterol to tissues and is directly atherogenic. Its levels correlate strongly with coronary artery disease risk. HDL cholesterol is inversely related to risk. Triglycerides and VLDL contribute indirectly. The LDL-C/HDL-C ratio provides a more precise cardiovascular risk index than total cholesterol alone.

Q141. Answer: B
Explanation: Metabolic alkalosis results from bicarbonate gain or acid loss (vomiting, diuretics). Both blood pH and bicarbonate rise, while pCO_2 increases as respiratory compensation. Decreased values indicate metabolic or respiratory acidosis. Distinguishing metabolic from respiratory causes depends on pCO_2 direction relative to pH and HCO_3^-.

Q142. Answer: B
Explanation: Aldosterone, secreted by the adrenal cortex, increases sodium reabsorption and potassium excretion in distal tubules, maintaining fluid balance and blood pressure. ADH regulates water only; renin initiates the renin-angiotensin-aldosterone cascade; cortisol affects metabolism. Aldosterone deficiency (Addison's disease) causes hyponatremia and hyperkalemia due to lost regulation.

Q143. Answer: B
Explanation: GGT is a microsomal enzyme elevated in hepatobiliary disorders and highly inducible by alcohol and drugs. It helps confirm hepatic source of alkaline phosphatase elevation. While ALT/AST rise in viral hepatitis, GGT elevation disproportionately high suggests chronic alcohol abuse or enzyme induction rather than acute hepatocellular injury.

Q144. Answer: C
Explanation: HbA1c reflects average blood glucose over 2-3 months, providing a long-term index of glycemic control and treatment effectiveness. Fasting glucose reflects short-term levels; OGTT diagnoses diabetes but not long-term control; fructosamine reflects 2-3 weeks. HbA1c remains gold standard for chronic glucose monitoring per ADA recommendations.

Q146. Answer: C
Explanation: ALT is predominantly located in hepatocytes and rises significantly with hepatocellular injury such as hepatitis or toxic damage. AST also elevates but is less specific due to presence in muscle and heart. ALP indicates cholestasis rather than hepatocellular necrosis. Lipase and CK elevations reflect pancreatic and muscle injury, respectively.

Q147. Answer: A
Explanation: In primary hypothyroidism, the thyroid gland fails to produce sufficient T_4, leading to feedback stimulation of TSH by the pituitary-thus high TSH and low T_4. Secondary hypothyroidism (pituitary failure) shows low TSH and T_4, while hyperthyroidism shows high T_4 with low TSH. TSH remains the most sensitive screening marker.

Q148. Answer: B
Explanation: BUN:creatinine ratio (>20:1) suggests prerenal azotemia due to reduced renal perfusion, while a normal ratio indicates intrinsic renal damage. Low ratios may occur in liver disease or

malnutrition. This ratio helps clinicians distinguish functional from structural kidney impairment quickly using routine chemistry tests.

Q149. Answer: A

Explanation: Arterial blood gas (ABG) analysis directly measures pH, pCO_2, and pO_2, allowing calculation of bicarbonate and base excess for comprehensive acid-base evaluation. Serum CO_2 approximates bicarbonate but lacks respiratory information. Urine pH reflects renal response, not systemic acid-base balance. ABG remains the diagnostic gold standard.

Q150. Answer: C

Explanation: Iron deficiency anemia presents with decreased serum iron and ferritin (storage), while total iron-binding capacity (TIBC) increases as the liver synthesizes more transferrin to capture available iron. This contrasts with anemia of chronic disease, where ferritin is high and TIBC low. The pattern differentiates nutritional deficiency from inflammation.

Q151. Answer: D

Explanation: Ammonia is detoxified in the liver via the urea cycle; hepatic dysfunction (e.g., cirrhosis, hepatitis) leads to accumulation causing encephalopathy. Renal failure increases urea, not ammonia. Diabetes and pancreatitis do not elevate ammonia significantly. Timely handling and chilled plasma collection are crucial since ammonia rapidly rises post-collection.

Q152. Answer: D

Explanation: Prostatic acid phosphatase (PAP) increases in prostate cancer, especially metastatic disease. However, prostate-specific antigen (PSA) is now preferred for screening and monitoring. ALP rises with bone metastases; ALT and GGT are liver markers. Historically, ACP helped confirm prostatic origin of metastasis prior to PSA assays.

Q153. Answer: D

Explanation: The bicarbonate-carbonic acid system is the principal extracellular buffer maintaining blood pH near 7.4. It reacts rapidly with metabolic acids and works in conjunction with respiratory CO_2 control. Hemoglobin and phosphate act as secondary buffers; plasma proteins contribute minimally. Bicarbonate's dynamic regulation by lungs and kidneys ensures stability.

Q154. Answer: C

Explanation: According to ADA criteria, diabetes mellitus is diagnosed with fasting glucose ≥126 mg/dL or 2-hour post-load glucose ≥200 mg/dL during OGTT. Normal values are <100 mg/dL fasting and <140 mg/dL post-load. Intermediate values indicate impaired glucose tolerance. Early diagnosis via these thresholds prevents complications through prompt management.

Q156. Answer: D

Explanation: HbA1c formation is proportional to mean blood glucose over RBC lifespan (120 days). High glucose promotes nonenzymatic hemoglobin glycation. RBC turnover inversely affects HbA1c; insulin levels do not directly influence it. Fructosamine reflects short-term glycation of serum proteins, not hemoglobin. HbA1c is the long-term index of glycemic control.

Q157. Answer: D

Explanation: Red cell rupture releases intracellular potassium and LDH, falsely elevating their serum levels. Sodium and chloride remain unaffected as extracellular ions. Calcium and phosphate may change minimally, while glucose and creatinine are stable. Proper specimen handling and prompt separation prevent hemolysis-related artifacts.

Q158. Answer: A

Explanation: CK-MB rises within 3-6 hours after myocardial infarction and peaks at 24 hours, preceding troponin elevation. Troponin is more specific but rises slightly later. LDH and AST elevate after 12-24 hours, remaining high for several days. Sequential CK-MB and troponin measurements confirm timing and progression of myocardial injury.

Q159. Answer: B

Explanation: Lactic acid forms under anaerobic conditions when oxygen delivery is insufficient, as in shock or hypoxia. Elevated lactate signals tissue hypoperfusion and metabolic acidosis. Aerobic metabolism consumes lactate; carbohydrate intake has minor influence. Measuring lactate assists in assessing oxygenation adequacy and sepsis severity.

Q161. Answer: D

Explanation: Hypernatremia typically arises from dehydration-water loss due to sweating, diabetes insipidus, or osmotic diuresis-rather than sodium gain. Addison's disease causes hyponatremia; SIADH leads to dilutional hyponatremia. Management focuses on gradual water replacement to avoid cerebral edema from rapid sodium correction.

Q162. Answer: B

Explanation: AST and ALT are aminotransferases released from damaged hepatocytes. Their isolated elevation signifies hepatocellular injury (viral hepatitis, toxins). Biliary obstruction increases ALP; bone disease affects ALP only. Mixed patterns occur in alcoholic cirrhosis with cholestasis. The ALT/AST ratio aids distinguishing alcoholic from viral hepatic injury.

Q163. Answer: C

Explanation: Excess insulin, either endogenous (insulinoma) or exogenous, drives glucose into cells, causing hypoglycemia. Adrenal insufficiency and liver disease may contribute but are less common. Thyrotoxicosis elevates, not lowers, glucose. Measuring insulin and C-peptide helps differentiate endogenous overproduction from external administration.

Q164. Answer: D

Explanation: Chylomicrons transport dietary triglycerides from intestines to tissues postprandially, giving plasma a milky appearance. They are cleared by lipoprotein lipase within hours. VLDL transports endogenous triglycerides; LDL and HDL primarily carry cholesterol. Fasting specimens eliminate chylomicron interference in lipid profiling.

Q166. Answer: A

Explanation: rosz: Uric acid derives from purine metabolism; elevated serum levels cause precipitation in joints (gout) or urine. Conditions with rapid cell turnover (leukemia, chemotherapy) increase uric acid production. Diabetes and infection affect glucose or WBCs, not uric acid. Identifying urate crystals supports gout or hyperuricemia diagnosis.

Q168. Answer: B

Explanation: The Jaffe reaction forms an orange-red complex between creatinine and alkaline picrate, used in creatinine assays. Biuret estimates total protein; Folin-Wu measures glucose; Van den Bergh quantifies bilirubin. Although widely used, Jaffe reaction may overestimate results due to interference from glucose and ketones unless corrected by enzymatic methods.

Q169. Answer: D

Explanation: Alkaline phosphatase (ALP) and GGT both rise in biliary obstruction. Elevated GGT confirms hepatic source since bone disease elevates ALP alone. AST/ALT remain normal, excluding hepatocellular injury. This pattern is characteristic of cholestatic disorders, allowing differentiation from bone pathology or muscle injury.

Q170. Answer: C

Explanation: Primary hyperparathyroidism increases PTH secretion, stimulating bone resorption and renal calcium reabsorption while enhancing phosphate excretion-resulting in high calcium and low phosphate. In malignancy-associated hypercalcemia, PTH is suppressed. Understanding PTH and phosphate dynamics is crucial for identifying endocrine versus non-endocrine causes of hypercalcemia.

Q171. Answer: A

Explanation: Gamma-glutamyl transferase (GGT) is highly inducible by alcohol and hepatotoxic drugs, showing marked elevation in alcoholic liver disease. ALT and AST increase in hepatocellular damage, but

GGT correlates best with chronic alcohol intake. ALP elevation suggests biliary obstruction. Persistent GGT elevation indicates enzyme induction from alcohol or medication exposure.

Q173. Answer: B

Explanation: Loss of bicarbonate through diarrhea or renal tubular acidosis reduces base without generating unmeasured anions, leading to a normal anion gap but elevated chloride (hyperchloremic acidosis). Lactic acidosis, ketoacidosis, and salicylate toxicity increase the anion gap instead. Identifying anion gap pattern aids in determining underlying mechanism.

Q174. Answer: A

Explanation: Cushing's syndrome features excessive cortisol secretion from adrenal tumors, hyperplasia, or exogenous steroids. Elevated cortisol suppresses ACTH in adrenal-origin disease but may remain high in pituitary-dependent (Cushing's disease). Aldosterone may be normal. Measuring cortisol after dexamethasone suppression distinguishes causes and confirms diagnosis.

Q176. Answer: C

Explanation: Microalbuminuria (30-300 mg/day) signifies early glomerular damage before overt proteinuria or renal function loss. Routine dipsticks lack sensitivity at this range. Serum creatinine and clearance rise later in disease. Detecting microalbumin allows timely glycemic and blood pressure control to prevent diabetic nephropathy progression.

Q178. Answer: D

Explanation: C-reactive protein rises dramatically in response to tissue injury, infection, or inflammation, serving as a sensitive acute-phase marker. Albumin and transferrin decrease during inflammation; prealbumin reflects nutritional status. Serial CRP monitoring helps track inflammatory activity and therapeutic response in autoimmune or infectious diseases.

Q179. Answer: A

Explanation: The estimated serum osmolality formula is $(2 \times Na^+) + (Glucose/18) + (BUN/2.8)$, expressing solutes in mmol/L. Sodium accounts for most osmotic activity; glucose and urea add smaller contributions. Comparing measured versus calculated osmolality reveals the osmolar gap, aiding toxic alcohol ingestion diagnosis or metabolic disturbance assessment.

Q180. Answer: D

Explanation: Adrenal medulla secretes catecholamines (epinephrine, norepinephrine); their metabolites metanephrines or vanillylmandelic acid (VMA) in urine diagnose pheochromocytoma. Cortisol and aldosterone assess adrenal cortex, not medulla. Renin activity pertains to renin-angiotensin system regulation. Elevated urinary metanephrines confirm catecholamine-producing tumors with high diagnostic specificity.

Q181. Answer: C

Explanation: During fasting, glycogen stores deplete, stimulating lipolysis and ketogenesis for energy. Free fatty acids and ketones rise while glucose and insulin decline. Amino acids provide gluconeogenic substrates but less significantly. Persistent ketosis indicates prolonged fasting or uncontrolled diabetes. Recognizing metabolic shifts prevents misinterpreting fasting hypoglycemia.

Q182. Answer: C

Explanation: Vitamin B_{12} deficiency impairs DNA synthesis, leading to megaloblastic anemia and neurologic defects. It uniquely elevates both homocysteine and methylmalonic acid. Folate deficiency elevates homocysteine only. Vitamin B_6 and niacin deficiencies cause other anemias or pellagra. Detecting B_{12} deficiency early prevents irreversible neurological damage.

Q183. Answer: D

Explanation: Hyperventilation reduces arterial CO_2, increasing pH and producing respiratory alkalosis. Anxiety, pain, or fever are common triggers. Hypoventilation and COPD cause CO_2 retention (acidosis). Metabolic acidosis involves bicarbonate loss, not respiratory origin. Correct diagnosis requires ABG correlation showing low pCO_2 with elevated pH.

Q184. Answer: B
Explanation: Primary hyperparathyroidism involves autonomous PTH secretion, elevating calcium by bone resorption and renal reabsorption. In malignancy, PTH decreases due to suppression; renal failure and vitamin D deficiency elevate PTH secondarily but calcium remains low or normal. Measuring both parameters distinguishes endocrine from reactive hyperparathyroid states.
Q185. Answer: C
Explanation: Lactate dehydrogenase (LDH) interconverts lactate and pyruvate with NAD^+/NADH as coenzyme. Its isoenzymes help localize tissue damage-LDH-1 and -2 (heart, RBCs) versus LDH-5 (liver, muscle). CK, ALT, and AST perform different metabolic reactions. LDH activity supports assessment of hemolysis, hepatic damage, and myocardial infarction.
Q186. Answer: A
Explanation: Addison's disease (primary adrenal insufficiency) causes reduced aldosterone and cortisol, leading to sodium loss (hyponatremia) and potassium retention (hyperkalemia). Water follows sodium loss, decreasing blood pressure. Opposite changes occur in hyperaldosteronism. Recognizing this electrolyte pattern confirms adrenal failure requiring corticosteroid and mineralocorticoid replacement therapy.
Q187. Answer: C
Explanation: Conjugated bilirubin rises in obstructive jaundice since bile cannot reach the intestine and regurgitates into plasma. Hemolytic anemia increases unconjugated bilirubin and urobilinogen from excessive RBC breakdown. LDH elevation occurs with hemolysis. Conjugated bilirubin's water solubility also results in bilirubinuria, distinguishing posthepatic obstruction from prehepatic causes.
Q188. Answer: A
Explanation: Cardiac troponins T and I are specific markers of myocardial injury, rising within hours after infarction and persisting for days. They surpass CK-MB in specificity and duration. Hepatic and renal tests use different analytes; muscular dystrophy elevates CK but not troponin. Troponins are now the gold standard for cardiac damage diagnosis.
Q189. Answer: B
Explanation: Alkaline phosphatase (ALP) originates from liver, bone, intestine, and placenta. Elevated ALP occurs in hepatic cholestasis and bone diseases (Paget's, metastases). GGT helps identify hepatic origin since it remains normal in bone disorders. ALT and LDH have different tissue sources. Isoenzyme analysis distinguishes ALP origin clinically.
Q192. Answer: B
Explanation: Chronic inflammation, autoimmune disorders, or infections stimulate immunoglobulin production, elevating the γ-globulin region on electrophoresis. Albumin typically decreases, α_1- and β-globulins may rise slightly. Polyclonal gammopathy signifies immune response, while monoclonal spikes suggest plasma cell dyscrasias like multiple myeloma. Electrophoresis differentiates reactive from neoplastic processes.
Q193. Answer: C
Explanation: Amylase and lipase both elevate in acute pancreatitis; lipase is more specific and remains elevated longer. Amylase can also rise in salivary disorders or perforated ulcers. ALT/AST relate to liver injury; CK/LDH to muscle; GGT/ALP to biliary tract. Simultaneous amylase and lipase rise strongly supports pancreatic inflammation.
Q194. Answer: B
Explanation: Alkaline phosphatase (ALP) rises markedly in cholestasis due to biliary epithelial enzyme induction. ALT and AST reflect hepatocellular damage, not bile obstruction. CK-MB indicates myocardial injury. When GGT is concurrently elevated, the hepatic origin of ALP increase is confirmed, ruling out bone-related causes.
Q195. Answer: D

Explanation: In primary hyperparathyroidism, PTH stimulates calcium release from bone and decreases renal phosphate reabsorption, resulting in hypercalcemia and hypophosphatemia. Hypoparathyroidism causes opposite changes. Vitamin D intoxication raises both calcium and phosphate; renal failure elevates phosphate with secondary hypocalcemia. The calcium-phosphate inverse pattern is diagnostic of parathyroid hyperfunction.

Q196. Answer: A

Explanation: The Guthrie test detects elevated phenylalanine levels in newborn blood using bacterial growth inhibition reversal. It screens for phenylketonuria caused by phenylalanine hydroxylase deficiency. Clinitest and Benedict's detect reducing sugars; Rothera's detects ketones. Early PKU detection allows dietary restriction to prevent neurological damage.

Q197. Answer: C

Explanation: Loss of gastric hydrochloric acid through vomiting or suction causes chloride and hydrogen depletion, producing metabolic alkalosis. Diarrhea leads to bicarbonate loss and metabolic acidosis. Salicylate toxicity initially causes respiratory alkalosis, then metabolic acidosis. Recognizing hypochloremic alkalosis guides fluid and chloride replacement therapy to restore acid-base balance.

Q199. Answer: A

Explanation: The glucose oxidase method specifically oxidizes glucose to gluconic acid and hydrogen peroxide, minimizing interference from other reducing substances. Benedict's, Clinitest, and copper-reduction tests react with any reducing sugar, giving false positives. Glucose oxidase's enzymatic specificity and automation suitability make it the reference method for clinical chemistry.

Q200. Answer: A

Explanation: Glucagon, secreted by pancreatic α-cells, elevates blood glucose by promoting glycogen breakdown and gluconeogenesis in the liver. Insulin lowers glucose by enhancing uptake and storage. Aldosterone regulates sodium, and calcitonin influences calcium metabolism. Glucagon's counter-regulatory role balances insulin to maintain glucose homeostasis, especially during fasting.

Question (201-300)

Q201. Which of the following is the primary site of hematopoiesis in an adult?

(A) Liver
(B) Lymph nodes
(C) Spleen
(D) Bone marrow

Q202. Erythropoietin (EPO) production increases primarily in response to:

(A) Tissue hypoxia
(B) Elevated blood pH
(C) Increased iron stores
(D) High plasma viscosity

Q203. Reticulocyte count provides information about:

(A) Coagulation function
(B) Bone marrow erythropoietic activity
(C) White cell maturity
(D) Platelet production rate

Q204. Which stain is used to identify reticulocytes?

(A) Sudan black B
(B) New methylene blue
(C) Wright-Giemsa
(D) Prussian blue

Q206. Anisocytosis refers to:

(A) Variation in cell size
(B) Nuclear fragmentation
(C) Cytoplasmic basophilia
(D) Variation in cell shape

Q207. Heinz bodies represent:

(A) Denatured hemoglobin precipitates
(B) Basophilic stippling
(C) RNA remnants
(D) Iron granules in RBCs

Q208. Basophilic stippling in RBCs is associated with:

(A) Megaloblastic anemia
(B) Lead poisoning or thalassemia
(C) Iron deficiency anemia
(D) Hemoglobin C disease

Q209. The mean corpuscular volume (MCV) indicates:

(A) Average red cell size
(B) Hemoglobin concentration per RBC
(C) Total hemoglobin content
(D) Variation in cell shape

Q210. Spherocytes are commonly associated with:

(A) Sickle cell trait
(B) Iron deficiency anemia
(C) Thalassemia minor
(D) Autoimmune hemolytic anemia

Q211. Target cells (codocytes) are most characteristic of:

(A) Aplastic anemia
(B) Megaloblastic anemia
(C) Iron deficiency anemia
(D) Thalassemia and liver disease

Q212. Sickle cells (drepanocytes) form due to:
(A) Vitamin deficiency
(B) Excess iron in RBCs
(C) Polymerization of hemoglobin S in deoxygenated state
(D) Oxidative hemoglobin denaturation

Q213. Howell-Jolly bodies are remnants of:
(A) RNA aggregates
(B) Denatured globin chains
(C) Nuclear DNA
(D) Iron granules

Q214. The prothrombin time (PT) evaluates which coagulation pathway?
(A) Common
(B) Fibrinolytic
(C) Extrinsic
(D) Intrinsic

Q215. The aPTT test evaluates the:
(A) Intrinsic and common pathways
(B) Fibrinogen concentration exclusively
(C) Extrinsic and common pathways
(D) Platelet function only

Q216. Mean corpuscular hemoglobin (MCH) reflects:
(A) Cell size variation
(B) Hemoglobin concentration per volume
(C) Total hemoglobin in blood
(D) Hemoglobin amount per red cell

Q217. Auer rods are diagnostic of:
(A) Acute lymphoblastic leukemia (ALL)
(B) Chronic lymphocytic leukemia (CLL)
(C) Acute myeloid leukemia (AML)
(D) Myelofibrosis

Q218. Which anticoagulant is used for routine hematology (CBC) testing?
(A) Sodium citrate
(B) Heparin
(C) EDTA (ethylenediaminetetraacetic acid)
(D) Oxalate

Q219. Left shift in neutrophils indicates:
(A) Presence of immature forms (bands, metamyelocytes) in circulation
(B) Reactive lymphocytosis
(C) Increase in lymphocytes
(D) Hyposegmentation of neutrophils

Q220. Hypersegmented neutrophils are characteristic of:
(A) Iron deficiency anemia
(B) Megaloblastic anemia
(C) Aplastic anemia

(D) Chronic myelogenous leukemia

Q221. Platelet satellitism occurs when platelets:

(A) Form clumps in heparin tubes

(B) Are excessively large due to marrow disorder

(C) Aggregate around neutrophils in EDTA-anticoagulated blood

(D) Adhere to glass surfaces

Q222. The primary function of platelets is to:

(A) Produce antibodies

(B) Transport oxygen

(C) Initiate hemostasis by forming plugs

(D) Regulate plasma volume

Q224. Hemoglobin electrophoresis identifies:

(A) Enzyme deficiencies

(B) Abnormal hemoglobin variants

(C) Leukocyte disorders

(D) Platelet defects

Q225. Reed-Sternberg cells are diagnostic of:

(A) Non-Hodgkin lymphoma

(B) Hodgkin lymphoma

(C) Chronic lymphocytic leukemia

(D) Multiple myeloma

Q226. Which of the following cells is the earliest recognizable erythroid precursor in the bone marrow?

(A) Polychromatophilic normoblast

(B) Reticulocyte

(C) Basophilic normoblast

(D) Pronormoblast

Q227. Myeloperoxidase (MPO) stain is used to differentiate:

(A) Platelets from megakaryocytes

(B) Plasma cells from lymphocytes

(C) Monocytes from macrophages

(D) Lymphoid from myeloid blasts

Q228. Pelger-Huët anomaly is characterized by:

(A) Toxic vacuolization

(B) Hyposegmented neutrophil nuclei

(C) Hypersegmented neutrophils

(D) Cytoplasmic granule deficiency

Q229. Toxic granulation and Döhle bodies in neutrophils are most often seen in:

(A) Bacterial infection or inflammation

(B) Leukemoid reaction

(C) Aplastic anemia

(D) Iron deficiency anemia

Q231. Hemoglobin H (β_4) is found in:

(A) α-thalassemia

(B) β-thalassemia

(C) Sickle cell anemia

(D) Hereditary spherocytosis

Q232. Elliptocytes (ovalocytes) are prominent in:

(A) Sickle cell anemia
(B) Hemolytic anemia of autoimmune origin
(C) Aplastic anemia
(D) Hereditary elliptocytosis

Q233. The Kleihauer-Betke test detects:
(A) Cold agglutinins
(B) Fetal hemoglobin in maternal circulation
(C) Heinz bodies
(D) Hemoglobin variants

Q234. Mean platelet volume (MPV) provides information on:
(A) Platelet size and marrow activity
(B) Platelet aggregation rate
(C) Clotting factor levels
(D) Hemoglobin synthesis

Q235. Plasma cell morphology includes:
(A) Nucleoli with basophilic cytoplasm
(B) Segmented nucleus with vacuoles
(C) Round eccentric nucleus and perinuclear halo
(D) Multilobed nucleus with granules

Q236. Teardrop cells (dacrocytes) are commonly seen in:
(A) Iron deficiency anemia
(B) Sickle cell anemia
(C) Hereditary spherocytosis
(D) Myelofibrosis

Q237. Smudge cells are characteristic of:
(A) Hodgkin lymphoma
(B) Megaloblastic anemia
(C) Chronic lymphocytic leukemia (CLL)
(D) Acute myeloid leukemia (AML)

Q238. The hemoglobin electrophoresis pattern in β-thalassemia minor typically shows:
(A) Increased HbS
(B) Normal HbA_2 and HbF
(C) Increased HbF only
(D) Increased HbA_2

Q239. G6PD deficiency leads to hemolysis primarily after:
(A) Viral infections
(B) Folate therapy
(C) Hypothermia
(D) Oxidative stress or certain drugs

Q240. Thrombocytopenia can result from all except:
(A) Immune destruction
(B) Increased erythropoietin production
(C) Decreased marrow production
(D) Splenic sequestration

Q241. Hyperleukocytosis (>100,000/µL) is most often seen in:
(A) Iron deficiency anemia
(B) Viral infection
(C) Megaloblastic anemia

(D) Leukemia

Q242. Disseminated intravascular coagulation (DIC) is characterized by:

(A) Normal D-dimer
(B) Increased fibrinogen
(C) Consumption of clotting factors and platelets
(D) Isolated thrombocytosis

Q243. Which RBC morphology is typical in iron deficiency anemia?

(A) Macrocytic, normochromic
(B) Microcytic, hypochromic
(C) Target cells
(D) Normocytic, normochromic

Q244. Sickle solubility test is used to detect:

(A) HbF concentration
(B) Leukemia cells
(C) RBC fragility
(D) Presence of hemoglobin S

Q245. Osmotic fragility test assesses:

(A) RBC membrane integrity
(B) Clotting factor activity
(C) Platelet function
(D) Hemoglobin concentration

Q247. Schistocytes on a blood smear are most associated with:

(A) Microangiopathic hemolytic anemia
(B) Aplastic anemia
(C) Thalassemia
(D) Iron deficiency anemia

Q248. Hemophilia A is caused by deficiency of:

(A) Factor XI
(B) Factor VIII
(C) Factor IX
(D) Factor X

Q249. Polycythemia vera is characterized by:

(A) Anemia with elevated EPO
(B) Low RBC mass, high EPO
(C) Normal hematocrit with high EPO
(D) Increased RBC mass, low EPO levels

Q250. Multiple myeloma is a malignancy of:

(A) B lymphocytes producing polyclonal antibodies
(B) T lymphocytes causing immune suppression
(C) Megakaryocytes overproducing platelets
(D) Plasma cells producing monoclonal immunoglobulin

Q251. Which stain is used to detect iron granules in red blood cells?

(A) New methylene blue
(B) Wright-Giemsa stain
(C) Sudan black B
(D) Prussian blue stain

Q252. Which condition presents with macrocytic, normochromic RBCs and hypersegmented neutrophils?

(A) Chronic renal failure
(B) Vitamin B12 or folate deficiency
(C) Thalassemia minor
(D) Iron deficiency anemia

Q253. Which white blood cell is primarily responsible for allergic reactions and parasitic defense?
(A) Monocyte
(B) Basophil
(C) Eosinophil
(D) Neutrophil

Q254. Döhle bodies consist of:
(A) RNA inclusions in neutrophils
(B) Denatured hemoglobin in RBCs
(C) DNA remnants in lymphocytes
(D) Iron granules in macrophages

Q255. Bence Jones proteins are:
(A) Ferritin-like proteins in plasma
(B) Fibrin degradation products
(C) Denatured albumin
(D) Free monoclonal light chains in urine

Q256. Hemoglobin F (fetal hemoglobin) differs from adult hemoglobin (HbA) by:
(A) Lacking heme groups
(B) Reduced oxygen affinity
(C) Containing δ-chains
(D) Having γ-chains instead of β-chains

Q257. Hereditary spherocytosis is caused by a defect in:
(A) Iron metabolism
(B) Hemoglobin synthesis
(C) Enzyme pathways
(D) RBC membrane proteins (spectrin, ankyrin)

Q258. Leukoerythroblastic reaction indicates:
(A) Elevated mature neutrophils
(B) Platelet clumping artifact
(C) Immature myeloid and nucleated RBCs in peripheral blood
(D) Pancytopenia

Q259. Disseminated intravascular coagulation (DIC) typically shows which laboratory pattern?
(A) Shortened PT, high platelets
(B) Prolonged PT and aPTT, low fibrinogen, elevated D-dimer
(C) Normal D-dimer, high fibrinogen
(D) Normal PT and aPTT, high fibrinogen

Q260. Hemoglobin electrophoresis is typically performed at what pH on cellulose acetate?
(A) 8.4
(B) 6.0
(C) 9.5
(D) 7.0

Q261. Myeloblasts can be identified by positive staining with:
(A) Periodic acid-Schiff (PAS)
(B) Alkaline phosphatase
(C) Myeloperoxidase (MPO) and Sudan black B

(D) Non-specific esterase

Q262. Which WBC abnormality is associated with infectious mononucleosis?

(A) Basophilia

(B) Monocytosis

(C) Neutrophilia

(D) Reactive lymphocytosis

Q263. Thalassemia major typically presents with:

(A) Severe microcytic anemia and target cells

(B) Macrocytic anemia and hypersegmented neutrophils

(C) Normocytic anemia with spherocytes

(D) Pancytopenia

Q264. Which coagulation factor is vitamin K-dependent?

(A) I, V, VIII, XIII

(B) Only factor VIII

(C) II, VII, IX, X

(D) XI, XII, prekallikrein, HMWK

Q265. Erythrocyte sedimentation rate (ESR) increases in:

(A) Dehydration

(B) Sickle cell disease

(C) Polycythemia

(D) Inflammation and infection

Q266. Burkitt lymphoma shows a classic "starry-sky" appearance due to:

(A) Fibrotic trabeculae

(B) Macrophages among proliferating lymphocytes

(C) Plasma cell clusters

(D) Necrotic neutrophils

Q267. Echinocytes (burr cells) are commonly associated with:

(A) Megaloblastic anemia

(B) Liver disease

(C) Uremia or artifact from excess EDTA

(D) G6PD deficiency

Q268. Acanthocytes (spur cells) are most characteristic of:

(A) Liver disease and abetalipoproteinemia

(B) Hemolytic anemia

(C) Iron deficiency anemia

(D) Thalassemia

Q269. Which white blood cell is mononuclear and capable of phagocytosis and antigen presentation?

(A) Monocyte

(B) Basophil

(C) Neutrophil

(D) Eosinophil

Q270. Factor XIII deficiency leads to:

(A) Normal PT and aPTT with delayed bleeding

(B) Prolonged PT and aPTT

(C) Isolated thrombocytopenia

(D) Elevated D-dimer

Q271. Chronic myeloid leukemia (CML) is associated with which chromosomal abnormality?

(A) t(8;14) translocation

(B) Philadelphia chromosome (t(9;22))
(C) Trisomy 21
(D) Deletion 13q
Q272. Which anticoagulant is used for coagulation studies such as PT and aPTT?
(A) Sodium citrate
(B) Heparin
(C) Fluoride oxalate
(D) EDTA
Q273. Neutrophilia with toxic granulation most likely indicates:
(A) Aplastic anemia
(B) Bacterial infection
(C) Leukemia
(D) Viral infection
Q274. LAP (leukocyte alkaline phosphatase) score is elevated in:
(A) Aplastic anemia
(B) Leukemoid reaction
(C) CML
(D) Acute leukemia
Q275. Hemoglobin C crystals appear in RBCs as:
(A) Needle-like rods
(B) Rhomboid or hexagonal dense inclusions
(C) Round Howell-Jolly bodies
(D) Basophilic stippling
Q276. Sickle cell disease can be confirmed by:
(A) ESR test
(B) Osmotic fragility test
(C) Hemoglobin electrophoresis
(D) Reticulocyte count
Q277. Absolute neutrophil count (ANC) below which level indicates severe neutropenia?
(A) $<2.0 \times 10^9/L$
(B) $<0.5 \times 10^9/L$
(C) $<1.5 \times 10^9/L$
(D) $<1.0 \times 10^9/L$
Q278. Hematocrit (Hct) represents:
(A) Oxygen saturation
(B) Hemoglobin concentration
(C) Percent of blood volume occupied by RBCs
(D) Plasma protein concentration
Q279. Megakaryocytes are responsible for producing:
(A) Erythrocytes
(B) Platelets
(C) Lymphocytes
(D) Monocytes
Q280. Cold agglutinin disease typically shows which lab artifact?
(A) Falsely increased MCV and decreased RBC count
(B) False thrombocytopenia
(C) Low MCV and high hemoglobin
(D) Decreased MCHC

Q281. Heinz bodies are best visualized with which stain?
(A) Crystal violet
(B) Wright-Giemsa
(C) Prussian blue
(D) Sudan black B
Q282. Bone marrow cellularity normally consists of:
(A) Entirely erythroid precursors
(B) 90% fat and 10% cells
(C) 50% hematopoietic cells and 50% fat in adults
(D) 75% lymphocytes
Q283. Hypochromia in RBCs indicates:
(A) Reduced hemoglobin content
(B) Increased cell volume
(C) Excess iron storage
(D) Vitamin deficiency
Q284. The Philadelphia chromosome (BCR-ABL) fusion gene activates:
(A) RNA polymerase
(B) Protein phosphatase
(C) DNA ligase
(D) Tyrosine kinase
Q285. Reticulocytosis typically occurs in:
(A) Bone marrow suppression
(B) Aplastic anemia
(C) Hemolytic anemia or blood loss
(D) Chronic renal failure
Q286. Sideroblastic anemia is caused by a defect in:
(A) Iron absorption
(B) Globin chain production
(C) Heme synthesis
(D) RBC membrane
Q287. Monospot test detects:
(A) Rheumatoid factor
(B) Heterophile antibodies
(C) Antinuclear antibodies
(D) Anti-dsDNA
Q288. Giant platelets are characteristic of:
(A) Von Willebrand disease
(B) Bernard-Soulier syndrome
(C) Glanzmann thrombasthenia
(D) Vitamin K deficiency
Q289. Roulette formation (rouleaux) occurs due to:
(A) Dehydration
(B) Vitamin deficiency
(C) Iron deficiency
(D) Increased plasma proteins (fibrinogen, globulins)
Q290. Tear drop cells (dacrocytes) on a peripheral smear most likely indicate:
(A) Lead poisoning
(B) Iron deficiency

(C) Vitamin C deficiency
(D) Bone marrow fibrosis or infiltration

Q291. Innate immunity differs from adaptive immunity by being:
(A) Induced by vaccination
(B) Non-specific and present at birth
(C) Antigen-specific and memory-based
(D) Mediated by lymphocytes only

Q292. The complement system enhances immunity by:
(A) Producing immunoglobulins
(B) Generating interferons
(C) Activating coagulation
(D) Lysing target cells via membrane attack complex

Q293. The classical complement pathway is initiated by:
(A) Mannose-binding lectin
(B) Antigen-antibody complexes
(C) C3 hydrolysis
(D) Bacterial endotoxins

Q294. $CD4^+$ T lymphocytes primarily function as:
(A) Cytotoxic cells killing infected cells
(B) Natural killer cells lysing tumor cells
(C) Suppressor cells reducing inflammation
(D) Helper cells activating B cells and macrophages

Q295. $CD8^+$ T lymphocytes are responsible for:
(A) Releasing histamine
(B) Producing antibodies
(C) Presenting antigen to B cells
(D) Directly killing virus-infected or tumor cells

Q296. Primary antibody response is characterized by:
(A) IgM production followed by IgG
(B) High-affinity IgA
(C) Absence of memory
(D) Immediate IgG secretion

Q298. The Western blot is used to confirm diagnosis of:
(A) Rheumatoid arthritis
(B) Syphilis
(C) Tuberculosis
(D) HIV infection

Q299. ELISA (enzyme-linked immunosorbent assay) detects:
(A) Complement activity
(B) Antigens or antibodies using enzyme-labeled conjugates
(C) Agglutination of RBCs
(D) Cellular immunity

Q300. Seroconversion refers to:
(A) Autoantibody suppression
(B) Development of detectable antibodies after infection or vaccination
(C) Loss of immune memory
(D) Change from IgM to IgA response

Answer Key and Explanation (201-300)

Q201. Answer: D

Explanation: In adults, bone marrow-particularly in the sternum, ribs, vertebrae, and pelvis-is the main site of hematopoiesis. The liver and spleen serve as extramedullary sites during fetal development or when marrow function is impaired. Lymph nodes are secondary lymphoid organs, supporting immune cell maturation but not primary hematopoiesis.

Q202. Answer: A

Explanation: Erythropoietin is produced by renal peritubular cells in response to tissue hypoxia. It stimulates erythroid progenitor proliferation and differentiation in bone marrow. Elevated iron or pH doesn't directly trigger EPO secretion. Chronic hypoxia or anemia therefore induces higher EPO levels, enhancing red blood cell production to improve oxygen delivery.

Q203. Answer: B

Explanation: Reticulocytes are immature RBCs containing residual RNA, reflecting recent marrow output. An elevated count signifies active erythropoiesis (e.g., hemolysis or blood loss), while low counts indicate marrow suppression or nutrient deficiency. They are stained with supravital dyes such as new methylene blue for enumeration under microscopy or flow cytometry.

Q204. Answer: B

Explanation: New methylene blue is a supravital stain that precipitates residual ribosomal RNA as a reticular network, identifying reticulocytes. Wright-Giemsa stains mature cell morphology, Prussian blue detects iron (siderocytes), and Sudan black B stains lipids in myeloid cells. Reticulocyte staining assists in assessing marrow response to anemia.

Q206. Answer: A

Explanation: Anisocytosis means unequal RBC sizes, often quantified by red cell distribution width (RDW). It is common in iron deficiency and mixed anemias. Poikilocytosis refers to abnormal shape variation. Recognizing anisocytosis assists in classifying anemia type and assessing red cell population heterogeneity from automated or microscopic findings.

Q207. Answer: A

Explanation: Heinz bodies are inclusions of denatured hemoglobin seen with oxidative damage, G6PD deficiency, or unstable hemoglobins. They require supravital stains (crystal violet or brilliant cresyl blue) for visualization. Iron granules form Pappenheimer bodies; RNA remnants produce basophilic stippling. Heinz body detection helps identify oxidative hemolysis disorders.

Q208. Answer: B

Explanation: Basophilic stippling results from precipitated ribosomal RNA, commonly seen in lead poisoning and thalassemia. It appears as fine to coarse blue granules dispersed throughout RBC cytoplasm on Wright stain. Iron deficiency anemia shows microcytosis without stippling, and megaloblastic anemia presents with macro-ovalocytes and hypersegmented neutrophils.

Q209. Answer: A

Explanation: MCV represents average RBC volume, calculated as (Hematocrit ÷ RBC count) × 10. It classifies anemia as microcytic, normocytic, or macrocytic. MCH indicates hemoglobin content per cell, while MCHC reflects hemoglobin concentration. MCV helps identify anemia etiology, such as microcytosis in iron deficiency or macrocytosis in B12 deficiency.

Q210. Answer: D

Explanation: Spherocytes are dense, spherical RBCs lacking central pallor due to membrane loss, typical of autoimmune hemolytic anemia and hereditary spherocytosis. Iron deficiency shows hypochromic microcytes; thalassemia minor has target cells; sickle trait yields occasional sickled forms. Spherocytosis causes increased osmotic fragility due to decreased surface-to-volume ratio.

Q211. Answer: D

Explanation: Target cells have increased membrane surface area relative to volume, forming a bull's-eye appearance. They occur in thalassemia (reduced hemoglobin synthesis) and liver disease (altered lipid composition). Iron deficiency anemia produces microcytosis without target formation; megaloblastic and aplastic anemias rarely show codocytes.

Q212. Answer: C

Explanation: In sickle cell disease, hemoglobin S polymerizes upon deoxygenation, distorting RBCs into sickle shapes. This causes vaso-occlusion and hemolysis. Oxidative denaturation produces Heinz bodies; iron overload forms siderocytes; vitamin deficiencies affect nuclear maturation. Sickle formation is reversible initially but becomes permanent with repeated deoxygenation cycles.

Q213. Answer: C

Explanation: Howell-Jolly bodies are small, round, basophilic nuclear DNA remnants in RBCs, often seen after splenectomy or in megaloblastic anemia. The spleen normally removes them from circulating cells. Pappenheimer bodies contain iron; basophilic stippling consists of RNA. Detection indicates asplenia or ineffective erythropoiesis with nuclear maturation defects.

Q214. Answer: C

Explanation: PT assesses the extrinsic and common coagulation pathways by measuring clotting time after adding tissue thromboplastin and calcium. It evaluates factors I (fibrinogen), II, V, VII, and X. Prolonged PT suggests factor VII deficiency, liver disease, or warfarin therapy. The intrinsic pathway is measured by activated partial thromboplastin time (aPTT).

Q215. Answer: A

Explanation: Activated partial thromboplastin time (aPTT) measures intrinsic and common coagulation pathways using phospholipid, activator, and calcium. It detects deficiencies in factors VIII, IX, XI, XII, and common pathway factors. Prolonged results occur in hemophilia, heparin therapy, or lupus anticoagulant. PT complements aPTT for comprehensive hemostasis assessment.

Q216. Answer: D

Explanation: MCH is the average weight of hemoglobin per RBC, calculated as (Hemoglobin ÷ RBC count) × 10. It helps classify anemia as hypochromic or normochromic. MCHC relates to hemoglobin concentration within cells, while MCV assesses size. Interpreting MCH with MCV aids in distinguishing iron deficiency from other anemias.

Q217. Answer: C

Explanation: Auer rods are azurophilic, needle-like inclusions of fused primary granules in myeloblasts, characteristic of acute myeloid leukemia, particularly the M2 and M3 (APL) subtypes. They are absent in lymphoid leukemias. Their presence confirms myeloid lineage in blasts and is important for diagnostic classification and treatment planning.

Q218. Answer: C

Explanation: EDTA is the preferred anticoagulant for complete blood count and differential studies because it preserves cellular morphology by chelating calcium. Citrate is used for coagulation testing; heparin for chemistry assays; oxalate for glucose preservation. Incorrect anticoagulant choice can alter cell integrity or interfere with automated counting.

Q219. Answer: A

Explanation: A left shift reflects increased immature neutrophil forms, commonly in bacterial infections or stress. It signals bone marrow stimulation and accelerated granulopoiesis. Lymphocytosis involves lymphoid cells, not neutrophils. Hyposegmentation (Pelger-Huët anomaly) is hereditary, not reactive. Left shift helps assess infection severity and marrow response.

Q220. Answer: B

Explanation: Hypersegmented neutrophils (≥6 lobes) are a hallmark of megaloblastic anemia due to vitamin B12 or folate deficiency. They reflect nuclear maturation delay caused by defective DNA synthesis. Iron deficiency and aplastic anemia show normal segmentation; CML presents with a full spectrum of myeloid precursors, not megaloblastic changes.

Q221. Answer: C

Explanation: Platelet satellitism is an EDTA-induced artifact where platelets adhere to neutrophils, causing falsely low automated platelet counts. It is corrected by recollecting in citrate. Heparin rarely causes this effect. Recognition under microscopy prevents misinterpretation of thrombocytopenia in laboratory results.

Q222. Answer: C

Explanation: Platelets initiate primary hemostasis by adhering to damaged endothelium, aggregating, and forming a platelet plug. They also provide a phospholipid surface for secondary coagulation. Oxygen transport is a red cell function; antibody production belongs to B lymphocytes. Platelet count and function testing evaluate bleeding disorders.

Q224. Answer: B

Explanation: Hemoglobin electrophoresis separates hemoglobin molecules based on charge and mobility, identifying variants such as HbS, HbC, HbF, or thalassemia patterns. Enzyme or leukocyte disorders require different assays. It's essential for diagnosing sickle cell disease and hemoglobinopathies through characteristic band migration on cellulose acetate or citrate agar media.

Q225. Answer: B

Explanation: Reed-Sternberg cells-large, binucleated cells with prominent nucleoli-are pathognomonic for Hodgkin lymphoma. They originate from B lymphocytes and are absent in non-Hodgkin types. CLL shows small mature lymphocytes; multiple myeloma features plasma cell proliferation. Identifying Reed-Sternberg morphology is crucial for lymphoma classification.

Q226. Answer: D

Explanation: The pronormoblast (rubriblast) is the earliest identifiable erythroid precursor, large with a prominent nucleus and deeply basophilic cytoplasm. It gives rise to basophilic normoblasts and eventually mature RBCs. Reticulocytes are non-nucleated late precursors released into circulation. Recognizing maturation stages is key in bone marrow morphology assessment.

Q227. Answer: D

Explanation: Myeloperoxidase stains primary granules of myeloid cells, helping distinguish myeloblasts (MPO positive) from lymphoblasts (MPO negative) in acute leukemias. It supports AML diagnosis versus ALL. Platelets, plasma cells, and monocytes have distinct cytochemical and immunophenotypic markers. MPO remains a fundamental cytochemical test in hematology.

Q228. Answer: B

Explanation: Pelger-Huët anomaly is a benign inherited condition featuring hyposegmented neutrophils (bilobed or dumbbell-shaped nuclei) with normal function. It must be distinguished from left shift or myelodysplasia. Hypersegmentation occurs in megaloblastic anemia, while toxic vacuolization reflects infection. Recognition prevents misinterpretation as pathologic immaturity.

Q229. Answer: A

Explanation: Toxic granulation and Döhle bodies indicate reactive changes in neutrophils due to severe bacterial infection or inflammation. Toxic granules are coarse azurophilic inclusions, and Döhle bodies are pale blue RNA remnants. They may also appear in pregnancy or chemotherapy. Recognizing these changes differentiates infection from neoplastic causes.

Q231. Answer: A

Explanation: Hemoglobin H (β_4 tetramers) forms in α-thalassemia when α-chain synthesis is reduced, leaving excess β-chains to aggregate. β-thalassemia involves decreased β-chain synthesis with increased HbA_2 or HbF. Sickle cell anemia produces HbS, and hereditary spherocytosis involves membrane defects, not hemoglobin structure abnormalities.

Q232. Answer: D

Explanation: Elliptocytes result from spectrin or protein 4.1 defects in hereditary elliptocytosis, causing elongated RBCs with normal hemoglobin. They may also appear in iron deficiency or thalassemia but less markedly. Sickle cells have crescent shapes; aplastic anemia shows normocytic cells with reduced count. Elliptocytes maintain normal osmotic fragility.

Q233. Answer: B

Explanation: The Kleihauer-Betke acid elution test identifies fetal RBCs containing HbF in maternal blood by staining them bright pink while adult cells appear ghost-like. It quantifies fetomaternal hemorrhage to guide Rh immune globulin dosing. Heinz bodies and hemoglobin variants require other specific stains or electrophoresis methods.

Q234. Answer: A

Explanation: MPV reflects average platelet size; larger platelets indicate increased marrow turnover or destruction (e.g., immune thrombocytopenia). Small platelets suggest production failure. MPV helps differentiate thrombocytopenia mechanisms. It is automatically calculated in CBCs, providing a rapid indirect assessment of megakaryocyte activity.

Q235. Answer: C

Explanation: Plasma cells are mature B cells with eccentric nuclei, clumped chromatin ("cartwheel pattern"), and perinuclear clearing (Golgi zone). They produce immunoglobulins and increase in chronic inflammation or multiple myeloma. Multilobed nuclei and granules characterize neutrophils; prominent nucleoli are blast features. Recognizing plasma cells aids immune disorder evaluation.

Q236. Answer: D

Explanation: Teardrop cells form when RBCs are squeezed out of fibrotic marrow, typical of myelofibrosis or marrow infiltration. They may accompany nucleated RBCs and immature myeloid forms (leukoerythroblastosis). Iron deficiency produces microcytosis, not teardrops. Dacrocytes are diagnostic clues to marrow fibrosis or infiltrative processes.

Q237. Answer: C

Explanation: Smudge cells are fragile lymphocytes that rupture during smear preparation, common in CLL due to cell membrane fragility. They appear as amorphous nuclear remnants. AML contains blasts with intact cytoplasm; Hodgkin lymphoma is tissue-based. Identifying smudge cells supports CLL diagnosis but may appear in other lymphoproliferative disorders.

Q238. Answer: D

Explanation: In β-thalassemia minor, decreased β-chain synthesis causes a compensatory rise in δ-chain production, increasing HbA_2 (>3.5%). HbF may be mildly elevated. HbS is absent unless co-inherited. Normal HbA_2 levels rule out β-thalassemia. Electrophoresis patterns are essential for distinguishing thalassemia from iron deficiency anemia.

Q239. Answer: D

Explanation: Glucose-6-phosphate dehydrogenase deficiency impairs RBC protection against oxidative damage, leading to hemolysis after exposure to drugs (sulfa, antimalarials), fava beans, or infections. Heinz bodies and bite cells appear microscopically. It's an X-linked disorder affecting red cell longevity. Avoiding oxidants prevents acute hemolytic episodes.

Q240. Answer: B

Explanation: Erythropoietin increases RBC production, not platelet destruction. Thrombocytopenia arises from immune causes (ITP), bone marrow failure, or hypersplenism. Identifying mechanism directs therapy-immunosuppression for immune causes, transfusion for aplasia, or splenectomy for sequestration. Platelet count and marrow evaluation confirm etiology.

Q241. Answer: D

Explanation: Extreme leukocytosis exceeding 100,000/μL typically indicates leukemia, especially CML or acute leukemias. Reactive infections rarely exceed 50,000/μL. Iron deficiency and megaloblastic anemias affect RBCs, not leukocyte counts. Recognizing marked leukocytosis triggers urgent evaluation for blast presence and potential leukostasis management.

Q242. Answer: C

Explanation: DIC involves systemic activation of coagulation, consuming platelets and factors, producing bleeding and microthrombi. Lab findings: prolonged PT/aPTT, low fibrinogen, elevated D-dimer, thrombocytopenia. It may occur secondary to sepsis, trauma, or malignancy. Rapid recognition and treating the underlying cause are crucial for survival.

Q243. Answer: B

Explanation: Iron deficiency anemia presents with microcytic, hypochromic RBCs due to inadequate hemoglobin synthesis. Peripheral smear shows small, pale cells with increased central pallor. Macrocytosis indicates vitamin B12/folate deficiency; target cells suggest thalassemia or liver disease. Microcytosis helps pinpoint iron-deficient states among anemias.

Q244. Answer: D

Explanation: The sickle solubility test uses a reducing agent that precipitates deoxygenated HbS, producing turbidity. It screens for HbS in sickle cell disease or trait. Hb electrophoresis confirms the result. HbF resists sickling; osmotic fragility tests assess membrane defects. The solubility test is quick but not quantitative.

Q245. Answer: A

Explanation: Osmotic fragility measures RBC resistance to hemolysis in hypotonic saline. Spherocytes (membrane loss) lyse early, while target cells resist lysis. It's used in hereditary spherocytosis diagnosis. Hemoglobin concentration and clotting activity require separate assays. This test evaluates the mechanical stability of erythrocyte membranes.

Q247. Answer: A

Explanation: Schistocytes (fragmented RBCs) occur from mechanical destruction in microangiopathic hemolytic anemia (MAHA), including DIC and TTP. Thalassemia and iron deficiency produce intact but small cells; aplastic anemia lacks abnormal shapes. Schistocyte detection indicates intravascular hemolysis and warrants urgent evaluation for thrombotic disorders.

Q248. Answer: B

Explanation: Hemophilia A results from factor VIII deficiency, inherited as an X-linked recessive disorder. Hemophilia B involves factor IX deficiency; both prolong aPTT with normal PT. Replacement therapy corrects clotting time. Recognition of specific factor deficiency guides targeted management and genetic counseling.

Q249. Answer: D

Explanation: Polycythemia vera is a myeloproliferative neoplasm with elevated RBC mass and suppressed EPO due to autonomous marrow proliferation (often JAK2 mutation). Secondary polycythemia arises from hypoxia or tumors with elevated EPO. High hematocrit and viscosity cause thrombosis risk, requiring phlebotomy and cytoreductive therapy.

Q250. Answer: D

Explanation: Multiple myeloma features clonal proliferation of plasma cells secreting monoclonal immunoglobulin (M protein). It causes bone lesions, hypercalcemia, renal failure, and anemia. Diagnosis includes serum protein electrophoresis, bone marrow biopsy, and Bence Jones protein detection. It differs from reactive plasmacytosis, which is polyclonal and benign.

Q251. Answer: D

Explanation: Prussian blue stain demonstrates ferric iron in RBCs and bone marrow cells, identifying sideroblasts and siderocytes. It is essential for diagnosing sideroblastic anemia and assessing iron stores. Wright-Giemsa stains cellular morphology; new methylene blue shows reticulocytes; Sudan black B identifies lipid granules in myeloid precursors.

Q252. Answer: B

Explanation: Vitamin B12 and folate deficiencies impair DNA synthesis, causing megaloblastic changes: macrocytic RBCs, hypersegmented neutrophils, and pancytopenia. Iron deficiency and thalassemia cause microcytosis, while renal failure leads to normocytic anemia. The peripheral smear and serum assays confirm the specific vitamin deficiency.

Q253. Answer: C

Explanation: Eosinophils combat parasitic infections and mediate allergic responses through histaminase and major basic protein release. Basophils release histamine but are fewer in number. Neutrophils handle bacterial infections, and monocytes become macrophages for phagocytosis. Eosinophilia commonly appears in allergy, asthma, and helminthic infestations.

Q254. Answer: A

Explanation: Döhle bodies are pale blue, oval inclusions composed of rough endoplasmic reticulum (RNA) found in neutrophils during infection, inflammation, or stress. They often accompany toxic granulation. Heinz bodies (denatured hemoglobin) and Howell-Jolly bodies (DNA) appear in RBCs, while iron granules form in macrophages and siderocytes.

Q255. Answer: D

Explanation: Bence Jones proteins are free κ or λ immunoglobulin light chains excreted in urine, produced by malignant plasma cells in multiple myeloma. They precipitate at 60°C and redissolve on boiling. Detection by electrophoresis or immunofixation confirms diagnosis. Ferritin, albumin, and fibrin fragments are unrelated protein types.

Q256. Answer: D

Explanation: HbF ($\alpha_2\gamma_2$) contains gamma chains instead of beta chains, allowing higher oxygen affinity for placental transfer. HbA ($\alpha_2\beta_2$) predominates in adults, and HbA_2 ($\alpha_2\delta_2$) forms a small portion. HbF is elevated in hereditary persistence and thalassemias. Its high affinity ensures fetal oxygenation even at low maternal oxygen tension.

Q257. Answer: D

Explanation: Hereditary spherocytosis results from defects in spectrin or ankyrin, disrupting membrane stability and causing spherical RBCs prone to splenic destruction. It presents with hemolytic anemia and increased osmotic fragility. Hemoglobinopathies involve synthesis defects, while enzyme deficiencies include G6PD or pyruvate kinase disorders.

Q258. Answer: C

Explanation: Leukoerythroblastic reaction shows immature myeloid cells and nucleated RBCs circulating, often due to marrow stress, fibrosis, or metastasis. It signals extramedullary hematopoiesis. Mature neutrophilia alone suggests infection, and pancytopenia reflects marrow suppression. Identifying both precursors on smear indicates bone marrow infiltration or extreme stimulation.

Q259. Answer: B

Explanation: DIC consumes clotting factors and platelets, prolonging PT/aPTT, reducing fibrinogen, and elevating D-dimer due to fibrin degradation. It results from sepsis, trauma, or malignancy. The combination of abnormal coagulation and thrombocytopenia confirms diagnosis. Management focuses on treating the cause and supportive replacement therapy.

Q260. Answer: A

Explanation: At alkaline pH (8.4), cellulose acetate electrophoresis separates hemoglobins by net charge. HbA migrates fastest toward the anode, followed by HbF, HbS, and HbC. Acid electrophoresis (pH 6.0-6.2) confirms ambiguous results by altering migration order. Dual-system testing ensures accurate hemoglobin variant identification.

Q261. Answer: C

Explanation: Myeloblasts contain primary granules positive for MPO and Sudan black B, distinguishing myeloid from lymphoid blasts. PAS stains lymphoblasts, while non-specific esterase marks monocytes.

Alkaline phosphatase assesses neutrophil activity. Cytochemical differentiation supports leukemia classification and treatment selection.

Q262. Answer: D

Explanation: Infectious mononucleosis from Epstein-Barr virus causes reactive lymphocytes-enlarged with abundant basophilic cytoplasm and indented nuclei. These cells are antigen-stimulated T lymphocytes. Neutrophilia suggests bacterial infection, while basophilia and monocytosis occur in allergic or chronic inflammatory states. Heterophile antibody (Monospot) confirms the diagnosis.

Q263. Answer: A

Explanation: Thalassemia major (Cooley's anemia) results from absent β-globin synthesis, producing severe microcytic, hypochromic anemia with target cells and nucleated RBCs. It manifests in infancy, requiring transfusion. Macrocytosis and hypersegmentation are megaloblastic features; spherocytes indicate membrane disorders. Diagnosis involves electrophoresis showing elevated HbF and HbA_2.

Q264. Answer: C

Explanation: Factors II, VII, IX, and X require vitamin K for γ-carboxylation, enabling calcium binding for clot formation. Warfarin inhibits this process, prolonging PT and aPTT. Deficiency causes bleeding due to impaired synthesis. Other factors like V, VIII, and XIII are not vitamin K-dependent.

Q265. Answer: D

Explanation: ESR rises during inflammation due to elevated fibrinogen and immunoglobulins promoting RBC aggregation (rouleaux formation). It decreases in polycythemia, dehydration, and sickle cell disease due to altered RBC morphology or reduced plasma proteins. ESR is a nonspecific marker of inflammation used to monitor chronic disease activity.

Q266. Answer: B

Explanation: Burkitt lymphoma features rapidly proliferating B cells interspersed with macrophages that engulf apoptotic debris, creating a "starry-sky" pattern microscopically. It is associated with Epstein-Barr virus and MYC translocation. Plasma cell and fibrotic patterns occur in other lymphoid neoplasms. Recognition aids diagnostic differentiation from other aggressive lymphomas.

Q267. Answer: C

Explanation: Echinocytes have short, uniform projections due to uremia or anticoagulant artifacts. Unlike acanthocytes (irregular spikes from liver disease), echinocytes are reversible. G6PD deficiency causes bite cells, and megaloblastic anemia shows macrocytosis. Proper smear preparation prevents artifactual burr cell formation.

Q268. Answer: A

Explanation: Acanthocytes have irregular spiculations from abnormal membrane lipid composition, commonly seen in liver disease and abetalipoproteinemia. Iron deficiency and thalassemia produce microcytosis, not spurs. These cells have reduced deformability, leading to splenic sequestration. Detection helps identify hepatic or lipid metabolic disorders.

Q269. Answer: A

Explanation: Monocytes are large mononuclear phagocytes that migrate into tissues to become macrophages, clearing debris and presenting antigens to lymphocytes. Neutrophils primarily phagocytose bacteria but lack antigen presentation. Eosinophils combat parasites; basophils mediate allergy. Monocyte counts rise in chronic infections and inflammation.

Q270. Answer: A

Explanation: Factor XIII stabilizes fibrin by cross-linking; its deficiency doesn't affect clot formation time, leaving PT and aPTT normal. However, clots are unstable and dissolve easily, causing delayed bleeding. It's rare and diagnosed via urea solubility tests. Recognition prevents misdiagnosis as platelet or coagulation disorder.

Q271. Answer: B

Explanation: CML involves the Philadelphia chromosome-reciprocal translocation between chromosomes 9 and 22-creating the BCR-ABL fusion gene, which increases tyrosine kinase activity. This mutation drives uncontrolled proliferation of myeloid cells. t(8;14) occurs in Burkitt lymphoma, while trisomy 21 relates to Down syndrome leukemias.

Q272. Answer: A

Explanation: Sodium citrate binds calcium reversibly, preserving factors for PT and aPTT assays. Correct 9:1 blood-to-anticoagulant ratio is essential. EDTA chelates calcium irreversibly, unsuitable for coagulation tests. Heparin is used for plasma chemistry, while fluoride oxalate inhibits glycolysis for glucose measurement.

Q273. Answer: B

Explanation: Bacterial infections stimulate bone marrow release of neutrophils, often with toxic granulation, Döhle bodies, and left shift. Viral infections produce lymphocytosis, leukemia shows abnormal blast forms, and aplastic anemia leads to pancytopenia. Recognizing neutrophilic response is key to identifying acute bacterial processes.

Q274. Answer: B

Explanation: The LAP score, reflecting neutrophil enzyme activity, is elevated in leukemoid reactions due to infection but decreased in CML due to defective cells. It remains normal in aplastic and acute leukemia. This distinction aids differentiation between reactive leukocytosis and myeloproliferative neoplasm.

Q275. Answer: B

Explanation: Hemoglobin C forms intracellular rhomboid or hexagonal crystals, especially after splenic removal. These dense inclusions distinguish HbC disease from HbS (sickle rods) and other inclusions. Basophilic stippling and Howell-Jolly bodies have different origins. Crystal detection supports hemoglobinopathy identification via microscopy and electrophoresis.

Q276. Answer: C

Explanation: Hemoglobin electrophoresis definitively identifies HbS in sickle cell disease, separating it from HbA, HbF, and HbC. Osmotic fragility and ESR are nonspecific, while reticulocyte count reflects marrow response, not diagnosis. Electrophoresis remains the confirmatory and quantitative method for hemoglobin variant identification.

Q277. Answer: B

Explanation: Severe neutropenia ($<0.5 \times 10^9$/L) greatly increases infection risk due to compromised innate immunity. Normal range is 1.5-8.0 $\times 10^9$/L. Moderate neutropenia (0.5-1.0) poses some risk, while mild (>1.0) is often asymptomatic. Identifying severity guides infection control and granulocyte colony-stimulating factor therapy.

Q278. Answer: C

Explanation: Hematocrit is the ratio of packed red blood cell volume to total blood volume, expressed as a percentage. It correlates with hemoglobin concentration and indicates anemia or polycythemia. Low hematocrit signifies anemia; high values indicate dehydration or erythrocytosis. It is routinely determined by automated analyzers or centrifugation.

Q279. Answer: B

Explanation: Megakaryocytes, large marrow cells, release cytoplasmic fragments called platelets into circulation. Each megakaryocyte produces thousands of platelets. Lymphocytes, monocytes, and erythrocytes derive from separate progenitors. Evaluating megakaryocyte morphology assists in diagnosing thrombocytopenia causes-reduced in marrow failure or increased in peripheral destruction.

Q280. Answer: A

Explanation: Cold agglutinins cause RBC clumping at low temperatures, leading to spuriously high MCV and low RBC count, thus elevating MCHC. Warming the specimen corrects these errors. The condition is associated with Mycoplasma infection or autoimmune hemolysis. Recognizing cold agglutination prevents misinterpretation of analyzer results.

Q281. Answer: A

Explanation: Heinz bodies, denatured hemoglobin inclusions, are visualized using supravital stains such as crystal violet or brilliant cresyl blue. They are not seen on Wright-Giemsa stains. These inclusions occur in G6PD deficiency or oxidative stress. Identifying Heinz bodies confirms oxidative hemolytic anemia etiology.

Q282. Answer: C

Explanation: Adult marrow is about 50% hematopoietic tissue and 50% fat, varying with age (rule of thumb: 100 minus age = % cellularity). Increased cellularity occurs in hyperplasia or leukemia; decreased in aplasia or chemotherapy. The erythroid-to-myeloid ratio and overall architecture are vital diagnostic indicators in marrow evaluation.

Q283. Answer: A

Explanation: Hypochromia refers to pale RBCs with increased central pallor, signifying low hemoglobin content, typically due to iron deficiency or thalassemia. Mean corpuscular hemoglobin concentration (MCHC) is reduced. Macrocytosis or vitamin deficiencies cause hyperchromic appearance. Detecting hypochromia assists in identifying hypoproliferative anemias.

Q284. Answer: D

Explanation: The BCR-ABL fusion gene, formed by t(9;22), encodes a constitutively active tyrosine kinase that drives uncontrolled cell proliferation in CML. Tyrosine kinase inhibitors (e.g., imatinib) target this abnormal activity. RNA polymerase and DNA ligase are unrelated enzymes. Identifying this mutation is diagnostic and therapeutic.

Q285. Answer: C

Explanation: Reticulocytosis reflects increased marrow response to RBC loss from hemolysis or hemorrhage. Reticulocytes are immature RBCs containing RNA remnants. Low counts indicate ineffective erythropoiesis as in aplastic anemia or renal EPO deficiency. Reticulocyte count is a vital index of marrow activity following anemia treatment.

Q286. Answer: C

Explanation: Sideroblastic anemia results from defective incorporation of iron into heme, producing ring sideroblasts in bone marrow. Causes include lead poisoning, alcoholism, and pyridoxine deficiency. Thalassemia affects globin chains; iron absorption disorders cause iron deficiency. Prussian blue staining confirms ring sideroblast presence.

Q287. Answer: B

Explanation: The Monospot test identifies heterophile antibodies produced during Epstein-Barr virus infection (infectious mononucleosis). These antibodies agglutinate horse or sheep RBCs. ANA and anti-dsDNA indicate lupus, while rheumatoid factor marks rheumatoid arthritis. The Monospot is a quick screening test for acute EBV infection.

Q288. Answer: B

Explanation: Bernard-Soulier syndrome features defective glycoprotein Ib, impairing platelet adhesion and producing large platelets. Von Willebrand disease affects factor VIII complex, not platelet size. Glanzmann thrombasthenia involves aggregation defects. Recognition of giant platelets with thrombocytopenia suggests inherited adhesion disorder.

Q289. Answer: D

Explanation: Rouleaux, the stacking of RBCs like coins, occurs when plasma proteins increase, reducing surface charge (zeta potential). It's seen in multiple myeloma and inflammation. Iron deficiency and vitamin deficiency affect size or color, not aggregation. Rouleaux elevates ESR and indicates altered plasma protein levels.

Q290. Answer: D

Explanation: Teardrop cells result from RBCs being squeezed out of fibrotic or infiltrated marrow, typical of myelofibrosis or metastatic infiltration. They appear alongside nucleated RBCs and leukoerythroblastosis. Iron deficiency causes microcytosis, and lead toxicity shows basophilic stippling. Dacrocytes signal distorted marrow architecture.

Q291. Answer: B

Explanation: Innate immunity provides the first line of defense, acting rapidly and non-specifically through physical barriers, complement, phagocytes, and natural killer cells. It lacks memory and specificity. Adaptive immunity, mediated by B and T lymphocytes, is antigen-specific and enhanced upon re-exposure. Innate mechanisms activate adaptive responses.

Q292. Answer: D

Explanation: Complement proteins form a cascade that opsonizes pathogens, promotes inflammation, and forms the membrane attack complex (C5b-C9) that lyses target cells. Immunoglobulins are produced by plasma cells, interferons by virally infected cells, and coagulation involves separate cascades. Complement bridges innate and adaptive immunity through antibody-mediated activation.

Q293. Answer: B

Explanation: The classical pathway begins when IgG or IgM binds antigen, activating C1 complex (C1q, C1r, C1s). The lectin pathway is triggered by mannose-binding lectin, while the alternative pathway starts with spontaneous C3 hydrolysis. Antibody-dependent complement activation links adaptive immunity to innate defense mechanisms.

Q294. Answer: D

Explanation: $CD4^+$ helper T cells orchestrate immune responses by releasing cytokines that activate B cells, macrophages, and cytotoxic T cells. $CD8^+$ T cells are cytotoxic; regulatory T cells suppress responses. NK cells are part of innate immunity. $CD4^+$ T-cell counts are critical indicators in HIV infection.

Q295. Answer: D

Explanation: $CD8^+$ cytotoxic T lymphocytes recognize antigen presented by MHC class I molecules on infected or abnormal cells and induce apoptosis through perforin and granzymes. B cells produce antibodies, and antigen presentation is performed by APCs. This response is central to adaptive cellular immunity against intracellular pathogens.

Q296. Answer: A

Explanation: During the first exposure, IgM is produced initially due to rapid pentameric formation, followed by class switching to IgG, which provides longer-lasting protection. Secondary responses yield faster and higher IgG titers due to memory cells. IgA functions in mucosal defense, not primary systemic response.

Q298. Answer: D

Explanation: Western blot detects HIV-specific antibodies against viral proteins separated by electrophoresis. It confirms reactive ELISA screening results. Syphilis uses treponemal tests (FTA-ABS), rheumatoid arthritis uses RF or anti-CCP assays, and tuberculosis is diagnosed via culture or interferon gamma release assays. Western blot ensures high specificity in HIV testing.

Q299. Answer: B

Explanation: ELISA employs enzyme-labeled antibodies or antigens that produce a measurable color reaction, detecting either antigen or antibody. It is widely used in infectious disease screening and hormone assays. Complement activity and cellular immunity require functional tests. ELISA's sensitivity and versatility make it a cornerstone of serologic testing.

Q300. Answer: B

Explanation: Seroconversion marks the transition from seronegative to seropositive status following infection or immunization when antibodies become detectable. It signifies adaptive immune activation. Class switching (IgM to IgG/IgA) occurs during the response but is distinct. Monitoring seroconversion confirms recent infection or effective vaccination.

Question (301-400)

Q301. Agglutination reactions involve:
(A) Particulate antigens and specific antibodies forming visible clumps
(B) Enzyme-substrate interactions
(C) Soluble antigens forming precipitation lines
(D) Radioactive labeling

Q302. Precipitation tests are best used for:
(A) Hemagglutinins
(B) Cellular antigens
(C) Soluble antigens
(D) Complement fixation

Q303. Autoimmune hemolytic anemia involves:
(A) Antibodies against bacterial proteins
(B) Complement deficiency
(C) Autoantibodies against self-RBC antigens
(D) Cytotoxic T-cell activation only

Q304. Rheumatoid factor (RF) is an antibody directed against:
(A) Complement component C3
(B) Histones
(C) DNA
(D) The Fc portion of IgG

Q305. Antinuclear antibody (ANA) testing is primarily used for diagnosing:
(A) Systemic lupus erythematosus (SLE)
(B) Celiac disease
(C) Multiple sclerosis
(D) Rheumatoid arthritis

Q306. Immunoglobulin class IgA is primarily found in:
(A) Serum only
(B) Complement system
(C) Secretions such as saliva, tears, and mucosa
(D) Cytotoxic T-cell membranes

Q307. An anamnestic response refers to:
(A) Nonspecific innate activation
(B) Initial IgM production only
(C) Delayed-type hypersensitivity
(D) Secondary immune response with rapid, high-affinity antibody production

Q308. Type I hypersensitivity is mediated by:
(A) Cytotoxic antibodies
(B) T-cell activation
(C) IgE and mast cell degranulation
(D) Immune complexes

Q309. Type II hypersensitivity includes:
(A) Anaphylaxis
(B) Hemolytic transfusion reactions
(C) Serum sickness
(D) Contact dermatitis

Q310. Type III hypersensitivity results from:

(A) Immune complex deposition in tissues
(B) Delayed inflammation
(C) IgE-mediated histamine release
(D) Cytotoxic T-cell destruction

Q311. Type IV hypersensitivity is primarily:
(A) T-cell-mediated delayed response
(B) Antibody-dependent complement activation
(C) IgE-mediated allergy
(D) Immediate hypersensitivity

Q312. HLA typing is important for:
(A) Organ transplantation compatibility
(B) Detecting autoimmune hemolysis
(C) Measuring complement function
(D) Identifying infections

Q313. Immunofluorescence assays (IFA) utilize:
(A) Enzyme-substrate color reactions
(B) Fluorescent-labeled antibodies for antigen detection
(C) Agglutination
(D) Radioactive isotopes

Q314. The prozone phenomenon occurs when:
(A) Complement activation fails
(B) Excess antibody prevents visible agglutination
(C) Excess antigen enhances precipitation
(D) Reagent contamination occurs

Q315. The indirect fluorescent antibody test (IFA) is used to detect:
(A) Complement levels
(B) Plasma proteins
(C) Direct antigen presence on cells
(D) Patient antibodies using labeled anti-human globulin

Q316. Titer in serologic testing refers to:
(A) The initial undiluted sample
(B) The highest dilution of serum that still gives a positive reaction
(C) The absolute concentration of antibody
(D) A qualitative measurement only

Q317. The rapid plasma reagin (RPR) test screens for:
(A) Syphilis
(B) HIV
(C) Rheumatic fever
(D) Hepatitis B

Q318. Complement fixation test (CFT) detects:
(A) Phagocytic function
(B) Free antigen by precipitation
(C) Antigen-antibody reactions based on complement consumption
(D) IgE-mediated allergy

Q319. Immunodeficiency due to HIV primarily affects:
(A) B lymphocytes
(B) Neutrophils
(C) $CD4^+$ T-helper lymphocytes

(D) NK cells

Q320. The main immunoglobulin crossing the placenta is:

(A) IgA

(B) IgM

(C) IgG

(D) IgE

Q321. Gram-positive cocci in clusters most likely indicate:

(A) Neisseria species

(B) Staphylococcus species

(C) Enterococcus species

(D) Streptococcus species

Q322. Which Staphylococcus species is coagulase positive?

(A) S. aureus

(B) S. saprophyticus

(C) S. epidermidis

(D) S. haemolyticus

Q323. Catalase test differentiates:

(A) E. coli from Salmonella

(B) Streptococcus from Enterococcus

(C) Staphylococcus (positive) from Streptococcus (negative)

(D) Neisseria from Moraxella

Q324. Alpha-hemolytic streptococci exhibit:

(A) Partial greenish hemolysis on blood agar

(B) Beta-hemolysis

(C) Clear complete hemolysis

(D) No hemolysis

Q325. Lancefield grouping classifies Streptococcus based on:

(A) Toxin production

(B) Hemolytic patterns

(C) Cell wall carbohydrate antigens

(D) Capsule composition

Q326. Group A Streptococcus (S. pyogenes) is sensitive to:

(A) Polymyxin B

(B) Bacitracin

(C) Optochin

(D) Novobiocin

Q327. Group B Streptococcus (S. agalactiae) causes:

(A) Rheumatic heart disease

(B) Strep throat

(C) Neonatal sepsis and meningitis

(D) Scarlet fever

Q328. Streptococcus pneumoniae appears as:

(A) Gram-negative rods

(B) Gram-negative diplococci

(C) Gram-positive, lancet-shaped diplococci

(D) Gram-positive cocci in clusters

Q329. Enterococcus faecalis is distinguished from Group D Streptococcus by:

(A) Growth in 6.5% NaCl broth

(B) Beta-hemolysis
(C) Optochin sensitivity
(D) Bacitracin resistance
Q330. Neisseria gonorrhoeae ferments which carbohydrate?
(A) Glucose only
(B) Glucose and maltose
(C) Lactose and maltose
(D) Sucrose only
Q331. Thayer-Martin medium is selective for:
(A) Salmonella species
(B) Staphylococcus aureus
(C) Neisseria gonorrhoeae and N. meningitidis
(D) E. coli
Q332. Enterobacteriaceae are characterized by:
(A) Spore-forming rods
(B) Gram-negative rods, oxidase negative, glucose fermenters
(C) Nonfermenting Gram-negative rods
(D) Gram-positive cocci, catalase positive
Q333. MacConkey agar differentiates bacteria based on:
(A) Oxygen utilization
(B) Spore formation
(C) Motility
(D) Lactose fermentation
Q334. Triple Sugar Iron (TSI) agar tests for:
(A) Capsule presence
(B) Protein synthesis
(C) Sugar fermentation and hydrogen sulfide production
(D) Lipase activity
Q335. Urease-positive bacteria include:
(A) E. coli
(B) Proteus species
(C) Shigella
(D) Salmonella
Q336. Motility test distinguishes:
(A) E. coli from Salmonella
(B) Klebsiella (nonmotile) from Enterobacter (motile)
(C) Shigella from Proteus
(D) Pseudomonas from Acinetobacter
Q337. Salmonella is differentiated from Shigella by:
(A) Lactose fermentation
(B) Gram stain morphology
(C) Catalase positivity
(D) H_2S production and motility
Q338. Campylobacter jejuni is best isolated at:
(A) 42°C in microaerophilic conditions
(B) 4°C in ambient air
(C) 25°C aerobically
(D) 37°C anaerobically

Q339. Vibrio cholerae causes disease through:
(A) Enterotoxin activating adenylate cyclase
(B) Endotoxin release causing sepsis
(C) Invasion of intestinal mucosa
(D) Neurotoxin-mediated paralysis
Q340. Pseudomonas aeruginosa is identified by:
(A) Lactose fermentation
(B) Blue-green pigment (pyocyanin) and fruity odor
(C) Gram-positive rods
(D) Catalase negativity
Q341. Legionella pneumophila requires which special medium for growth?
(A) EMB agar
(B) MacConkey agar
(C) Buffered charcoal yeast extract (BCYE) agar
(D) Blood agar
Q342. Clostridium tetani produces a toxin that:
(A) Induces watery diarrhea
(B) Blocks inhibitory neurotransmitters, causing spastic paralysis
(C) Causes flaccid paralysis
(D) Destroys neutrophils
Q343. Clostridium difficile infection is associated with:
(A) Antibiotic therapy disrupting normal flora
(B) Poor water sanitation
(C) Ingestion of contaminated meat
(D) Mosquito bites
Q344. Mycobacterium tuberculosis is best identified by:
(A) Gram stain
(B) Acid-fast staining (Ziehl-Neelsen)
(C) India ink preparation
(D) Silver stain
Q345. Mycobacterium tuberculosis transmission occurs primarily by:
(A) Vector bites
(B) Inhalation of airborne droplets
(C) Skin contact
(D) Fecal-oral route
Q346. Mycobacterium tuberculosis grows best on which medium?
(A) MacConkey agar
(B) Blood agar
(C) EMB agar
(D) Lowenstein-Jensen medium
Q347. Acid-fast bacteria resist decolorization due to:
(A) Spore coats
(B) Peptidoglycan layer only
(C) Capsule polysaccharides
(D) Mycolic acid in the cell wall
Q348. Mycobacterium leprae causes:
(A) Anthrax
(B) Hansen’s disease (leprosy)

(C) Tuberculosis
(D) Diphtheria
Q349. Corynebacterium diphtheriae produces a toxin that:
(A) Destroys myelin sheaths
(B) Stimulates excessive cAMP
(C) Inhibits protein synthesis via EF-2 inactivation
(D) Causes hemolysis
Q350. Listeria monocytogenes is distinguished by:
(A) Nonmotility
(B) Beta-hemolysis absence
(C) Tumbling motility at room temperature
(D) Catalase negativity
Q351. Bacillus anthracis forms:
(A) Motile rods with capsules
(B) Small Gram-negative cocci
(C) Acid-fast filaments
(D) Large, nonmotile, spore-forming Gram-positive rods
Q352. Clostridium botulinum toxin causes:
(A) Spastic paralysis
(B) Diarrhea by cAMP activation
(C) Hemolytic anemia
(D) Flaccid paralysis by blocking acetylcholine release
Q353. Clostridium perfringens is associated with:
(A) Diphtheria-like illness
(B) Pseudomembranous colitis
(C) Lockjaw
(D) Gas gangrene and food poisoning
Q354. Haemophilus influenzae requires which factors for growth?
(A) X (hemin) and V (NAD) factors
(B) Only V factor
(C) Only X factor
(D) None
Q355. Bordetella pertussis causes:
(A) Pneumonic plague
(B) Diphtheria
(C) Scarlet fever
(D) Whooping cough
Q356. Bordetella pertussis virulence is mainly due to:
(A) Pertussis toxin and tracheal cytotoxin
(B) Capsule polysaccharide
(C) Flagellar antigens
(D) Lipid A endotoxin only
Q357. Klebsiella pneumoniae is known for:
(A) Swarming motility
(B) Noncapsulated dry colonies
(C) Oxidase positivity
(D) Thick polysaccharide capsule and mucoid colonies
Q358. Escherichia coli O157:H7 is associated with:

(A) Hemolytic uremic syndrome (HUS)
(B) Dysentery by invasion
(C) Typhoid fever
(D) Cholera-like diarrhea
Q359. Salmonella Typhi infection primarily spreads through:
(A) Airborne droplets
(B) Vector bites
(C) Blood transfusion
(D) Fecal-oral route via contaminated food or water
Q360. Shigella dysenteriae produces a toxin that:
(A) Inhibits protein synthesis by inactivating 60S ribosomes
(B) Causes hemolysis
(C) Increases cAMP secretion
(D) Blocks acetylcholine
Q361. Yersinia pestis causes:
(A) Typhoid
(B) Plague
(C) Cholera
(D) Tetanus
Q362. Helicobacter pylori infection is diagnosed by:
(A) Acid-fast stain
(B) Throat culture
(C) Urease breath test or biopsy urease activity
(D) Gram stain of stool
Q363. Treponema pallidum is best visualized by:
(A) Dark-field microscopy
(B) Acid-fast stain
(C) Gram staining
(D) India ink preparation
Q364. Borrelia burgdorferi causes:
(A) Syphilis
(B) Lyme disease
(C) Rocky Mountain spotted fever
(D) Relapsing fever
Q365. Leptospira interrogans infection is acquired by:
(A) Inhalation of droplets
(B) Contact with urine of infected animals
(C) Tick bites
(D) Sexual transmission
Q366. Rickettsia rickettsii causes:
(A) Lyme disease
(B) Q fever
(C) Rocky Mountain spotted fever
(D) Typhus
Q367. Chlamydia trachomatis causes:
(A) Tuberculosis
(B) Gonorrhea
(C) Nongonococcal urethritis and trachoma

(D) Syphilis

Q368. Mycoplasma pneumoniae lacks:

(A) A cell wall
(B) DNA
(C) Ribosomes
(D) Plasma membrane

Q369. Candida albicans forms:

(A) Yeast, pseudohyphae, and germ tubes
(B) Only spores
(C) Encapsulated cocci
(D) Acid-fast rods

Q370. Cryptococcus neoformans is identified by:

(A) Acid-fast staining
(B) Hyphal morphology
(C) India ink preparation showing encapsulated yeasts
(D) Germ tube test

Q371. Aspergillus fumigatus commonly causes:

(A) Oral thrush
(B) Pneumocystis pneumonia
(C) Pulmonary aspergillosis
(D) Cryptococcal meningitis

Q372. Zygomycetes (Mucor, Rhizopus) infections are associated with:

(A) Tetanus
(B) Tuberculosis
(C) Hepatitis
(D) Diabetic ketoacidosis

Q373. Pneumocystis jirovecii pneumonia is diagnosed by:

(A) India ink test
(B) Silver stain of lung specimens showing cysts
(C) Gram stain
(D) Acid-fast staining

Q374. Histoplasma capsulatum infection is associated with:

(A) Vector transmission
(B) Skin penetration
(C) Inhalation of bat or bird droppings
(D) Ingestion of contaminated food

Q375. Blastomyces dermatitidis is a:

(A) Dimorphic fungus causing pulmonary and skin disease
(B) Bacterium
(C) Protozoan parasite
(D) Yeast causing vaginitis

Q376. Coccidioides immitis causes:

(A) Valley fever (coccidioidomycosis)
(B) Histoplasmosis
(C) Aspergillosis
(D) Blastomycosis

Q377. Toxoplasma gondii infection is transmitted through:

(A) Blood transfusion

(B) Ingestion of oocysts from cat feces or undercooked meat
(C) Airborne droplets
(D) Mosquito bites

Q378. Plasmodium falciparum infection is transmitted by:
(A) Female Anopheles mosquito bite
(B) Tsetse fly
(C) Tick
(D) Sandfly

Q379. Babesia microti infection resembles malaria but is transmitted by:
(A) Ixodes ticks
(B) Fleas
(C) Mosquitoes
(D) Mites

Q380. Trypanosoma brucei causes:
(A) Amebiasis
(B) African sleeping sickness
(C) Chagas disease
(D) Leishmaniasis

Q381. Trypanosoma cruzi infection is acquired via:
(A) Airborne spores
(B) Feces of reduviid (kissing) bugs entering bite wounds
(C) Contaminated food
(D) Mosquito bites

Q382. Leishmania donovani causes:
(A) Trypanosomiasis
(B) Filariasis
(C) Malaria
(D) Visceral leishmaniasis (kala-azar)

Q383. Entamoeba histolytica infection results in:
(A) Amoebic dysentery and liver abscess
(B) Trichomoniasis
(C) Giardiasis
(D) Malaria

Q384. Giardia lamblia infection is characterized by:
(A) CNS infection
(B) Bloody diarrhea
(C) Greasy, foul-smelling stools and malabsorption
(D) Urethritis

Q385. Trichomonas vaginalis is identified by:
(A) Silver stain
(B) Motile trophozoites on wet mount
(C) Acid-fast stain
(D) Cysts in stool

Q386. Taenia saginata infection results from:
(A) Ingestion of undercooked beef containing cysticerci
(B) Contaminated vegetables
(C) Undercooked pork
(D) Fish ingestion

Q387. Taenia solium causes:
(A) Anemia due to blood loss
(B) Only intestinal infection
(C) Cutaneous disease
(D) Cysticercosis when eggs are ingested
Q388. Echinococcus granulosus infection produces:
(A) Hydatid cysts in liver and lungs
(B) Hookworm disease
(C) Malaria
(D) Trichinosis
Q389. Enterobius vermicularis (pinworm) diagnosis uses:
(A) ELISA antigen test
(B) Blood culture
(C) Stool acid-fast stain
(D) Cellophane tape test for perianal eggs
Q390. Schistosoma haematobium infection primarily affects the:
(A) Intestine
(B) Urinary bladder
(C) Lungs
(D) Liver
Q391. Quality control (QC) in the clinical laboratory ensures:
(A) Increased test volume only
(B) Accuracy and reliability of test results
(C) Reduced reagent usage
(D) Administrative record keeping only
Q392. Proficiency testing (PT) is designed to:
(A) Calibrate instruments
(B) Train laboratory personnel
(C) Evaluate laboratory performance using external unknown samples
(D) Validate new test methods
Q393. Levey-Jennings charts are used to:
(A) Monitor QC data over time for trends or shifts
(B) Document staff attendance
(C) Record reagent inventory
(D) Schedule instrument maintenance
Q394. Westgard rules help:
(A) Detect analytical errors using statistical QC limits
(B) Measure turnaround time
(C) Set reagent expiration dates
(D) Document personnel competency
Q395. Preventive maintenance in laboratories aims to:
(A) Reduce instrument downtime and ensure performance reliability
(B) Eliminate calibration needs
(C) Increase test cost
(D) Replace instruments regularly
Q396. Chain of custody documentation is required in:
(A) Serology screening
(B) Blood typing only

(C) Routine chemistry testing
(D) Forensic or legal specimen handling

Q397. The Occupational Safety and Health Administration (OSHA) primarily regulates:

(A) Laboratory worker safety and hazardous exposure control
(B) Laboratory accreditation
(C) Patient data confidentiality
(D) Test billing procedures

Q398. Biological safety cabinets (BSC) protect:

(A) Only personnel
(B) Personnel, environment, and specimen from contamination
(C) Only the environment
(D) Only the specimen

Q399. Standard precautions require:

(A) Wearing PPE only for known infections
(B) Using gloves for sterile samples only
(C) Handwashing only after visible contamination
(D) Treating all specimens as potentially infectious

Q400. Root cause analysis (RCA) is used for:

(A) Investigating errors to identify underlying system causes
(B) Reviewing normal QC data
(C) Repeating patient tests for confirmation
(D) Validating new instruments

Answer Key and Explanation (301-400)

Q301. Answer: A

Explanation: Agglutination occurs when particulate antigens (cells, beads) interact with antibodies, forming visible clumps. It's used in blood typing and bacterial identification. Precipitation involves soluble antigens, enzyme reactions define ELISA, and radioimmunoassays use radiolabels. Agglutination tests demonstrate antibody-antigen recognition in a direct, visual manner.

Q302. Answer: C

Explanation: Precipitation occurs when soluble antigen and antibody combine in optimal proportions to form insoluble complexes. Examples include immunodiffusion and immunoelectrophoresis. Cellular antigens cause agglutination instead, while hemagglutinins cause RBC clumping. Precipitation helps detect antigenic relationships and measure antibody concentration.

Q303. Answer: C

Explanation: In autoimmune hemolytic anemia, IgG or IgM autoantibodies bind self-RBCs, causing complement-mediated or extravascular destruction. It may be idiopathic or secondary to lupus or drugs. Direct antiglobulin testing confirms RBC-bound antibodies. Complement deficiency causes infection susceptibility, not hemolysis.

Q304. Answer: D

Explanation: Rheumatoid factor is an IgM antibody targeting the Fc portion of IgG, forming immune complexes that deposit in joints, causing inflammation. It's characteristic of rheumatoid arthritis but may appear in infections or other autoimmune diseases. Anti-CCP testing offers greater specificity for rheumatoid arthritis diagnosis.

Q305. Answer: A

Explanation: ANA testing detects antibodies against nuclear components, commonly positive in systemic lupus erythematosus and other connective tissue diseases. Pattern analysis (homogeneous, speckled, nucleolar) provides diagnostic clues. Rheumatoid arthritis involves RF; multiple sclerosis and celiac disease use different antibody markers. ANA remains the hallmark lupus screen.

Q306. Answer: C

Explanation: IgA protects mucosal surfaces by neutralizing pathogens in saliva, tears, respiratory, and gastrointestinal secretions. It exists as a dimer linked by J chain and secretory component. Serum IgA plays a minor role compared to secretory IgA. It is crucial in mucosal immunity, preventing pathogen adherence.

Q307. Answer: D

Explanation: An anamnestic response is the secondary, memory-driven immune response producing high-titer, high-affinity IgG rapidly upon re-exposure to the same antigen. It reflects immunologic memory from prior infection or vaccination. Delayed-type hypersensitivity is cell-mediated; innate responses lack specificity. This mechanism underlies booster immunization effectiveness.

Q308. Answer: C

Explanation: Type I (immediate) hypersensitivity involves IgE binding to mast cells and basophils, triggering histamine release upon re-exposure to allergen-manifesting as hay fever, asthma, or anaphylaxis. Type II is cytotoxic (IgG/IgM), Type III immune complex-mediated, and Type IV cell-mediated (delayed). Type I reactions occur within minutes.

Q309. Answer: B

Explanation: Type II hypersensitivity involves IgG or IgM antibodies binding to cell-surface antigens, activating complement, and causing cell lysis, as seen in hemolytic transfusion reactions or hemolytic disease of the newborn. Serum sickness (Type III) involves immune complexes, contact dermatitis (Type IV) is T-cell-mediated, and anaphylaxis is Type I.

Q310. Answer: A

Explanation: Type III reactions occur when antigen-antibody complexes deposit in tissues, activating complement and causing inflammation (e.g., serum sickness, lupus nephritis). Type I involves IgE, Type II cytotoxic antibodies, and Type IV delayed-type T-cell responses. Immune complex pathology leads to vasculitis and glomerulonephritis.

Q311. Answer: A

Explanation: Type IV hypersensitivity (delayed-type) involves sensitized T cells releasing cytokines that recruit macrophages, leading to tissue inflammation 24-72 hours after exposure (e.g., tuberculin reaction, contact dermatitis). It does not involve antibodies. Recognizing this mechanism explains delayed immune responses in skin testing and transplant rejection.

Q312. Answer: A

Explanation: Human leukocyte antigen (HLA) typing matches donor and recipient tissues to minimize graft rejection, particularly for kidney and bone marrow transplants. It also aids disease association studies (e.g., HLA-B27 and ankylosing spondylitis). It's unrelated to complement assays or infection identification.

Q313. Answer: B

Explanation: IFA uses fluorochrome-labeled antibodies that bind specific antigens, visualized under a fluorescence microscope. It's used for detecting autoantibodies (e.g., ANA) and infectious agents. ELISA employs enzyme reactions; RIA uses radioisotopes; agglutination involves visible clumping. IFAs provide sensitive and specific antigen localization.

Q314. Answer: B

Explanation: In prozone effect, antibody excess interferes with lattice formation, yielding false-negative agglutination. Diluting the sample restores optimal antigen-antibody ratio. Antigen excess causes postzone effect. Recognizing prozone prevents misinterpretation of tests like syphilis RPR or ASO titers, ensuring accurate serologic results.

Q315. Answer: D

Explanation: Indirect IFA detects patient antibodies bound to known antigens by adding fluorescent-labeled anti-human globulin. The direct method labels antibodies bound directly to antigen. Complement assays and protein quantification require different techniques. Indirect IFA is widely applied in autoimmune and infectious disease serology.

Q316. Answer: B

Explanation: Titer represents the highest serum dilution showing a visible positive reaction in serologic assays, reflecting antibody strength. It provides a semiquantitative measure of immune response. A higher titer indicates greater antibody concentration. This measure aids in diagnosis, disease monitoring, and immunity assessment after infection or vaccination.

Q317. Answer: A

Explanation: RPR detects reagin antibodies against cardiolipin-lecithin antigen, screening for syphilis. It's a non-treponemal test used for initial diagnosis and monitoring therapy. Confirmatory testing uses treponemal assays (FTA-ABS or TP-PA). HIV and hepatitis require separate antibody or antigen tests, while rheumatic fever relies on ASO titers.

Q318. Answer: C

Explanation: CFT determines presence of antigen or antibody by measuring complement consumption during immune complex formation. If complement is fixed, no hemolysis occurs in indicator cells-signifying a positive result. It's used for historical viral and fungal serology. Other tests detect allergies, precipitation, or cellular immunity.

Q319. Answer: C

Explanation: HIV targets $CD4^+$ T-helper cells via gp120 binding, causing depletion and immune collapse. This loss impairs both humoral and cellular responses, leading to opportunistic infections and malignancies. B cells, NK cells, and neutrophils remain functionally secondary targets. CD4 count monitoring reflects disease progression and antiretroviral therapy efficacy.

Q320. Answer: C

Explanation: IgG, the smallest and most abundant immunoglobulin, crosses the placenta via Fc receptor-mediated transport, providing passive immunity to the fetus. IgM, being large, cannot cross; its presence in neonates indicates intrauterine infection. IgA and IgE are primarily mucosal and allergic antibodies, respectively. Maternal IgG protects infants postnatally.

Q321. Answer: B

Explanation: Staphylococcus species appear as Gram-positive cocci in clusters, resembling grapes under microscopy. Streptococcus and Enterococcus form chains or pairs, while Neisseria are Gram-negative diplococci. Catalase positivity differentiates Staphylococcus from Streptococcus, which is catalase negative. This morphology guides initial identification of bacterial isolates.

Q322. Answer: A

Explanation: S. aureus produces coagulase, converting fibrinogen to fibrin, forming clots that protect bacteria from phagocytosis. S. epidermidis and S. saprophyticus are coagulase negative. The coagulase test distinguishes pathogenic S. aureus from less virulent staphylococci, confirming infection in abscesses, pneumonia, or bacteremia.

Q323. Answer: C

Explanation: Catalase test detects enzyme breakdown of hydrogen peroxide into water and oxygen, forming bubbles. Staphylococcus species are catalase positive, while Streptococcus and Enterococcus are negative. This simple test provides the first differential step among Gram-positive cocci during routine bacterial identification.

Q324. Answer: A

Explanation: Alpha-hemolytic streptococci partially lyse RBCs, producing a green zone on blood agar due to methemoglobin formation. Streptococcus pneumoniae and viridans group are examples. Beta-hemolytic strains (e.g., S. pyogenes) cause clear zones, while gamma-hemolytic species show none. Hemolytic pattern aids classification of streptococci.

Q325. Answer: C

Explanation: Lancefield grouping identifies Streptococcus species by cell wall carbohydrate antigens (Groups A-H, K-V). S. pyogenes is Group A, S. agalactiae Group B, and Enterococcus Group D. Hemolytic patterns provide preliminary grouping, but antigenic classification confirms species. This system aids diagnosis of streptococcal infections.

Q326. Answer: B

Explanation: Group A S. pyogenes shows zone of inhibition around bacitracin disc on blood agar, distinguishing it from other β-hemolytic streptococci. S. pneumoniae is optochin sensitive, S. saprophyticus is novobiocin resistant, and polymyxin B is used against Gram-negative bacteria. Bacitracin screening remains a quick presumptive test.

Q327. Answer: C

Explanation: S. agalactiae colonizes maternal genital tract and transmits to neonates during birth, leading to sepsis and meningitis. S. pyogenes causes pharyngitis and scarlet fever; rheumatic fever follows untreated infections. Screening pregnant women and intrapartum prophylaxis effectively prevent neonatal infections by Group B Streptococcus.

Q328. Answer: C

Explanation: S. pneumoniae are Gram-positive, lancet-shaped diplococci exhibiting alpha-hemolysis and optochin sensitivity. Their polysaccharide capsule is the major virulence factor. Neisseria species are Gram-negative diplococci, while Staphylococcus forms clusters. Proper identification is vital since S. pneumoniae causes pneumonia, meningitis, and otitis media.

Q329. Answer: A

Explanation: Enterococcus faecalis grows in 6.5% NaCl and hydrolyzes bile esculin, unlike nonenterococcal Group D Streptococcus bovis. It causes urinary, wound, and endocardial infections. Hemolysis pattern varies, and it's resistant to many antibiotics. Growth in high salt concentration is a key differentiating feature.

Q330. Answer: A

Explanation: N. gonorrhoeae ferments glucose but not maltose, lactose, or sucrose. N. meningitidis ferments glucose and maltose. This biochemical distinction aids identification. Gram-negative intracellular diplococci in urethral exudate confirm gonorrhea. Culture on Thayer-Martin medium and nucleic acid amplification tests provide definitive diagnosis.

Q331. Answer: C

Explanation: Thayer-Martin agar contains antibiotics (vancomycin, colistin, nystatin) that inhibit contaminants, allowing Neisseria gonorrhoeae and N. meningitidis to grow. S. aureus and E. coli are suppressed. This selective medium is essential for isolating pathogenic Neisseria from mixed clinical specimens such as genital or throat swabs.

Q332. Answer: B

Explanation: Enterobacteriaceae are Gram-negative, non-spore-forming rods that ferment glucose and are oxidase negative. Members include E. coli, Klebsiella, Proteus, and Salmonella. Nonfermenters like Pseudomonas are oxidase positive. This family includes normal flora and major pathogens of the intestinal tract, urinary tract, and bloodstream.

Q333. Answer: D

Explanation: MacConkey agar contains bile salts and crystal violet to inhibit Gram-positive growth and differentiates lactose fermenters (pink colonies, e.g., E. coli) from nonfermenters (colorless colonies, e.g., Salmonella). It's both selective and differential for Gram-negative enteric bacteria, crucial in stool and urine cultures.

Q334. Answer: C

Explanation: TSI agar contains glucose, lactose, sucrose, and iron salts to detect fermentation and H_2S production. Blackening indicates H_2S; yellow slants/butts denote acid production. It differentiates enteric bacteria-Salmonella produces H_2S, Shigella does not. This test is key for presumptive identification in stool isolates.

Q335. Answer: B

Explanation: Proteus species produce urease, hydrolyzing urea into ammonia and CO_2, raising pH. This reaction differentiates Proteus from Salmonella and Shigella, which are urease negative. Rapid urease activity contributes to urinary stone formation. Urease test aids identification of urease-positive pathogens like Proteus and Helicobacter pylori.

Q336. Answer: B

Explanation: Klebsiella species are nonmotile due to lack of flagella, while Enterobacter are motile. Both are lactose fermenters and can appear similar on MacConkey agar. Motility testing differentiates them and other enteric organisms. This distinction aids in identifying urinary and respiratory pathogens accurately.

Q337. Answer: D

Explanation: Salmonella produces H_2S and is motile, while Shigella is nonmotile and H_2S negative. Both are non-lactose fermenters on MacConkey agar. These features distinguish enteric pathogens causing gastroenteritis and dysentery. Confirmatory serotyping follows biochemical screening for accurate identification.

Q338. Answer: A

Explanation: C. jejuni thrives at 42°C in microaerophilic atmosphere (5% O_2, 10% CO_2), reflecting adaptation to avian hosts. It causes bacterial gastroenteritis, typically from undercooked poultry.

Isolation requires selective media like Campy-BAP. Its curved, motile, Gram-negative rods and darting motility aid recognition.

Q339. Answer: A

Explanation: Cholera toxin activates adenylate cyclase in intestinal cells, increasing cAMP, leading to chloride and water secretion-causing profuse watery diarrhea. It does not invade mucosa. Endotoxin-related sepsis occurs in other Gram-negative infections, while neurotoxins are characteristic of Clostridium species.

Q340. Answer: B

Explanation: Pseudomonas aeruginosa produces blue-green pigment (pyocyanin) and emits a fruity odor, key traits alongside oxidase positivity and nonfermentative metabolism. It causes opportunistic infections in burns, cystic fibrosis, and immunocompromised patients. Its antibiotic resistance and biofilm formation make it clinically challenging to treat.

Q341. Answer: C

Explanation: Legionella pneumophila grows on BCYE agar enriched with L-cysteine and iron, essential for its metabolism. It does not grow on standard media. This organism causes Legionnaires' disease, acquired via inhalation of aerosolized water sources. Direct fluorescent antibody and PCR aid rapid detection.

Q342. Answer: B

Explanation: Tetanospasmin, produced by C. tetani, inhibits release of glycine and GABA from inhibitory neurons, causing sustained muscle contraction (spastic paralysis). C. botulinum causes flaccid paralysis; C. perfringens induces gas gangrene; C. difficile causes colitis. Vaccination with toxoid prevents tetanus effectively.

Q343. Answer: A

Explanation: Antibiotic use suppresses normal intestinal flora, allowing C. difficile overgrowth and toxin production, leading to pseudomembranous colitis. Common culprits include clindamycin and broad-spectrum antibiotics. Diagnosis uses stool toxin assays or PCR. Proper antibiotic stewardship and infection control reduce incidence.

Q344. Answer: B

Explanation: M. tuberculosis retains carbol fuchsin dye after acid-alcohol decolorization due to high lipid content (mycolic acids) in its cell wall. Ziehl-Neelsen and fluorescent auramine-rhodamine stains are diagnostic. It resists Gram staining and grows slowly on Lowenstein-Jensen medium, requiring biosafety precautions.

Q345. Answer: B

Explanation: Tuberculosis spreads via airborne droplet nuclei expelled by coughing or sneezing. The bacilli infect alveolar macrophages and form granulomas. Fecal-oral and vector routes are not involved. Airborne isolation and early detection are critical for prevention, especially in healthcare environments.

Q346. Answer: D

Explanation: Lowenstein-Jensen medium, containing malachite green, provides nutrients and inhibits contaminants, supporting slow growth of M. tuberculosis. Colonies appear rough, buff-colored after 2-8 weeks. MacConkey and EMB select for Gram-negative organisms, and blood agar supports most fast growers but not acid-fast bacilli. LJ medium is diagnostic standard.

Q347. Answer: D

Explanation: Mycolic acids in the waxy cell wall of acid-fast bacteria, like Mycobacterium and Nocardia, retain carbol fuchsin despite acid-alcohol treatment. This lipid barrier resists staining by conventional dyes and chemical injury. The acid-fast property is key for identification of these pathogens in clinical samples.

Q348. Answer: B

Explanation: M. leprae causes Hansen's disease, affecting skin and peripheral nerves. It cannot be cultured on artificial media and is diagnosed by acid-fast bacilli in skin smears or biopsy. M. tuberculosis causes pulmonary TB; Bacillus anthracis causes anthrax; Corynebacterium diphtheriae causes diphtheria. Early detection prevents disability.

Q349. Answer: C

Explanation: The diphtheria toxin inhibits host cell protein synthesis by inactivating elongation factor-2 (EF-2), leading to pseudomembrane formation in the throat. The toxin gene is phage-encoded. Other pathogens like Vibrio cholerae increase cAMP, while neurotoxins affect nerves. Diphtheria vaccination provides effective protection via toxoid.

Q350. Answer: C

Explanation: Listeria monocytogenes exhibits tumbling motility at 25°C and shows beta-hemolysis on blood agar. It's a facultative intracellular pathogen causing neonatal sepsis and meningitis, often from unpasteurized foods. Catalase positivity and cold enrichment growth further aid identification. Differentiating Listeria prevents perinatal infections.

Q351. Answer: D

Explanation: Bacillus anthracis is a large, nonmotile, spore-forming Gram-positive rod with a unique poly-D-glutamate capsule. It causes anthrax, manifesting as cutaneous, inhalational, or gastrointestinal disease. Nonpathogenic Bacillus species are motile and lack capsules. Endospore formation contributes to environmental persistence and infection potential.

Q352. Answer: D

Explanation: The botulinum toxin prevents acetylcholine release at neuromuscular junctions, producing flaccid paralysis and respiratory failure. C. tetani toxin causes spastic paralysis; C. perfringens affects tissues via alpha toxin. Botulism arises from improperly preserved foods. Heat-labile toxin and antitoxin therapy are crucial in management.

Q353. Answer: D

Explanation: C. perfringens causes gas gangrene through alpha toxin (lecithinase) that destroys tissues and RBCs. It also causes food poisoning via enterotoxin in contaminated meat. C. difficile causes colitis, C. tetani lockjaw, and C. diphtheriae pseudomembranes. Gram-positive, spore-forming rods confirm diagnosis microscopically.

Q354. Answer: A

Explanation: Haemophilus influenzae requires both X (hemin) and V (NAD) factors, found in chocolate agar but not blood agar. Satellitism near S. aureus colonies occurs due to released NAD. H. parainfluenzae requires only V factor. Recognition of factor requirements aids accurate differentiation within Haemophilus species.

Q355. Answer: D

Explanation: Bordetella pertussis infects ciliated respiratory epithelium, producing toxins that cause paroxysmal coughing fits ("whooping cough"). Diagnosis relies on nasopharyngeal swabs cultured on Bordet-Gengou or Regan-Lowe medium and PCR. Vaccination (DTaP) prevents disease. Diphtheria and plague involve different bacteria and mechanisms.

Q356. Answer: A

Explanation: Pertussis toxin increases cAMP, impairing immune cell function, while tracheal cytotoxin damages ciliated epithelial cells. Together they cause characteristic cough and lymphocytosis. Endotoxin and capsule contribute minimally. These virulence factors explain severe respiratory symptoms and underscore vaccine importance in preventing pertussis.

Q357. Answer: D

Explanation: Klebsiella pneumoniae produces large, mucoid colonies due to its thick capsule, which enhances virulence and antibiotic resistance. It causes pneumonia, UTIs, and sepsis, particularly in immunocompromised hosts. Proteus exhibits swarming, and Pseudomonas is oxidase positive. Capsule visualization is key for identification.

Q358. Answer: A

Explanation: EHEC E. coli O157:H7 produces Shiga-like toxin, damaging renal endothelium, causing HUS characterized by anemia, thrombocytopenia, and renal failure. It's transmitted via undercooked beef or unpasteurized juice. Unlike Shigella, it's noninvasive. Identified by sorbitol-nonfermenting colonies on SMAC agar.

Q359. Answer: D

Explanation: Salmonella Typhi, the causative agent of typhoid fever, spreads by ingestion of contaminated food or water. It invades intestinal mucosa and disseminates systemically. Transmission prevention includes sanitation and vaccination. Airborne and vector routes are not involved in typhoid epidemiology.

Q360. Answer: A

Explanation: Shiga toxin cleaves rRNA of the 60S ribosomal subunit, halting protein synthesis, leading to mucosal damage and bloody diarrhea. It's similar to E. coli O157:H7 toxin. Vibrio cholerae increases cAMP; Clostridium toxins affect nerves or membranes. Shiga toxin contributes to dysentery's severity.

Q361. Answer: B

Explanation: Yersinia pestis, transmitted via flea bites or aerosols, causes bubonic, septicemic, or pneumonic plague. Bipolar-staining "safety pin" appearance aids diagnosis. It's a zoonotic pathogen maintained in rodent reservoirs. Rapid antibiotic therapy and vector control prevent outbreaks. Other diseases involve distinct enteric or spore-forming pathogens.

Q362. Answer: C

Explanation: H. pylori produces urease, detectable in urea breath tests or biopsy CLO tests. It colonizes gastric mucosa, causing gastritis and ulcers. Gram stain of stool and acid-fast stains are irrelevant. Eradication requires antibiotic combination and acid suppression to prevent peptic ulcer recurrence.

Q363. Answer: A

Explanation: Treponema pallidum, the causative agent of syphilis, is too thin for Gram staining and is best observed by dark-field microscopy. Serologic tests (VDRL, FTA-ABS) confirm diagnosis. Acid-fast and India ink stains are used for other pathogens. Early identification aids treatment and prevents transmission.

Q364. Answer: B

Explanation: Borrelia burgdorferi, transmitted by Ixodes ticks, causes Lyme disease, presenting with erythema migrans and systemic symptoms. Diagnosis involves serologic ELISA and Western blot. Borrelia recurrentis causes relapsing fever; Rickettsia rickettsii causes spotted fever. Tick avoidance and prompt removal prevent infection.

Q365. Answer: B

Explanation: Leptospirosis results from exposure to water contaminated by urine of infected animals, entering via skin abrasions or mucosa. It causes fever, jaundice, and renal failure (Weil's disease). Zoonotic but not vector-borne, it's common in tropical regions. Preventive measures include protective clothing and sanitation.

Q366. Answer: C

Explanation: R. rickettsii, transmitted by tick bites, infects endothelial cells, causing vasculitis and characteristic rash of Rocky Mountain spotted fever. Typhus is caused by R. prowazekii, Q fever by Coxiella burnetii. Early doxycycline therapy prevents severe complications. Diagnosis relies on serology and clinical presentation.

Q367. Answer: C

Explanation: C. trachomatis causes ocular trachoma and sexually transmitted nongonococcal urethritis. It's an obligate intracellular pathogen detected by NAAT. Syphilis (Treponema pallidum) and gonorrhea

(Neisseria gonorrhoeae) have distinct etiologies. Treatment with azithromycin or doxycycline effectively eradicates infection and prevents chronic complications.

Q368. Answer: A

Explanation: Mycoplasma pneumoniae lacks a cell wall, rendering it resistant to beta-lactam antibiotics. It adheres to respiratory epithelium, causing atypical pneumonia ("walking pneumonia"). It contains sterols in its membrane for stability. Diagnosis uses cold agglutinins and molecular tests. Macrolides or tetracyclines are preferred treatments.

Q369. Answer: A

Explanation: Candida albicans exhibits yeast, pseudohyphae, and germ tubes (in serum at 37°C), diagnostic of infection. It causes thrush, vaginitis, and systemic candidiasis in immunocompromised hosts. Germ tube test rapidly distinguishes C. albicans from other yeasts. Acid-fastness and encapsulation do not apply to fungi.

Q370. Answer: C

Explanation: Cryptococcus neoformans possesses a thick polysaccharide capsule visible as a halo in India ink preparations of CSF. It causes cryptococcal meningitis, especially in immunocompromised patients. Confirmed by cryptococcal antigen test or culture on Sabouraud agar. Germ tube test and hyphae characterize Candida, not Cryptococcus.

Q371. Answer: C

Explanation: Aspergillus fumigatus produces airborne spores that infect lungs, causing aspergilloma or invasive aspergillosis in immunocompromised hosts. Candida causes thrush, Cryptococcus meningitis, and Pneumocystis jirovecii pneumonia in AIDS patients. Septate hyphae branching at 45° angles and fruiting heads confirm Aspergillus infection microscopically.

Q372. Answer: D

Explanation: Mucormycosis caused by Rhizopus and Mucor occurs mainly in diabetic ketoacidosis or immunosuppression. These fungi invade blood vessels, causing tissue necrosis and black nasal eschars. Broad, nonseptate hyphae distinguish them from Aspergillus. Rapid antifungal treatment and surgical debridement are life-saving in mucormycosis.

Q373. Answer: B

Explanation: Pneumocystis jirovecii (formerly P. carinii) causes pneumonia in AIDS and immunosuppressed patients. Cysts are visualized by Gomori methenamine silver or toluidine blue stains. It does not stain with Gram or acid-fast methods. Diagnosis can also be confirmed via PCR or immunofluorescence. Trimethoprim-sulfamethoxazole is treatment of choice.

Q374. Answer: C

Explanation: Histoplasma capsulatum spores found in bird and bat droppings are inhaled, causing pulmonary infection mimicking tuberculosis. It's endemic in the Ohio and Mississippi River valleys. It's a dimorphic fungus-mold in environment, yeast in tissues. Diagnosis involves histopathology or antigen detection in urine or serum.

Q375. Answer: A

Explanation: Blastomyces dermatitidis is a dimorphic fungus existing as mold in the environment and as thick-walled yeast with broad-based buds in tissues. It causes pulmonary and cutaneous infections in North America. Candida causes vaginitis; protozoa and bacteria are unrelated. Fungal culture and microscopy confirm diagnosis.

Q376. Answer: A

Explanation: Coccidioides immitis, endemic to the southwestern U.S., produces arthroconidia that, when inhaled, form spherules containing endospores in lungs. This causes Valley fever, which can disseminate in immunocompromised hosts. It's a dimorphic fungus. Differentiation from Histoplasma and Blastomyces is based on morphology and geographic location.

Q377. Answer: B

Explanation: Toxoplasma gondii spreads via ingestion of oocysts from cat feces or tissue cysts in undercooked meat. Congenital infection causes severe fetal abnormalities. Diagnosis is by serology or PCR. Immunocompromised patients risk encephalitis. Proper hygiene and avoiding raw meat prevent toxoplasmosis.

Q378. Answer: A

Explanation: Malaria caused by Plasmodium falciparum is transmitted through bites of infected Anopheles mosquitoes. The parasite infects RBCs, leading to hemolysis and anemia. Tsetse flies transmit trypanosomiasis; sandflies transmit leishmaniasis; ticks transmit babesiosis. Blood smear showing multiple ring forms per RBC supports P. falciparum diagnosis.

Q379. Answer: A

Explanation: Babesia microti, a protozoan parasite transmitted by Ixodes ticks, infects RBCs, causing babesiosis with hemolytic anemia. It mimics malaria microscopically but lacks pigment and gametocytes. Maltese cross formations in RBCs are diagnostic. Co-infection with Borrelia burgdorferi (Lyme disease) may occur in endemic regions.

Q380. Answer: B

Explanation: Trypanosoma brucei, transmitted by tsetse flies, causes African sleeping sickness, characterized by fever, lymphadenopathy, and CNS involvement leading to somnolence. T. cruzi causes Chagas disease; Leishmania causes leishmaniasis. Trypomastigotes in blood smear confirm infection. Control focuses on vector eradication and early antiparasitic therapy.

Q381. Answer: B

Explanation: T. cruzi causes Chagas disease, transmitted when feces of reduviid bugs enter bite wounds. Chronic infection causes cardiomyopathy and megacolon. Blood smear reveals trypomastigotes; amastigotes appear in tissue biopsy. Prevention includes insect control and improved housing in endemic Latin American areas.

Q382. Answer: D

Explanation: Leishmania donovani, transmitted by sandfly bites, causes visceral leishmaniasis characterized by fever, hepatosplenomegaly, and pancytopenia. Amastigotes (Leishman-Donovan bodies) are seen in macrophages from bone marrow or spleen. Other Leishmania species cause cutaneous or mucocutaneous disease. Vector control reduces transmission.

Q383. Answer: A

Explanation: Entamoeba histolytica causes amoebic dysentery with bloody diarrhea and hepatic abscesses due to tissue invasion. Cysts and trophozoites with ingested RBCs are diagnostic in stool. Giardia lamblia causes greasy stools; Trichomonas vaginalis affects genital tract. Proper sanitation and water filtration prevent transmission.

Q384. Answer: C

Explanation: Giardia lamblia attaches to intestinal mucosa via ventral adhesive disc, causing malabsorption, bloating, and steatorrhea. Cysts transmitted via contaminated water are resistant to chlorine. Diagnosis uses stool antigen or microscopic cyst detection. It's common among campers and travelers, treated with metronidazole.

Q385. Answer: B

Explanation: T. vaginalis exists only as motile trophozoites, visible under wet mount microscopy with jerky motion. It causes vaginitis and urethritis, transmitted sexually. No cyst form exists. Gram or acid-fast stains are unnecessary. Rapid antigen and nucleic acid tests also confirm infection.

Q386. Answer: A

Explanation: Taenia saginata (beef tapeworm) infection occurs after ingesting cysticerci in undercooked beef. T. solium (pork tapeworm) causes cysticercosis when eggs are ingested. Eggs and proglottids in stool confirm diagnosis. Proper meat inspection and thorough cooking prevent tapeworm infections.

Q387. Answer: D

Explanation: Ingestion of T. solium eggs leads to cysticercosis, where larvae invade tissues, including the brain (neurocysticercosis). Eating undercooked pork causes intestinal tapeworm infection. Diagnosis includes imaging and serology. Preventive measures focus on sanitation, proper pork cooking, and avoiding fecal contamination.

Q388. Answer: A

Explanation: Echinococcus granulosus larvae form hydatid cysts in human organs after accidental ingestion of eggs from dog feces. Cysts contain protoscolices and can rupture, causing anaphylaxis. Surgical removal and albendazole therapy are treatment options. Control involves deworming dogs and proper livestock handling.

Q389. Answer: D

Explanation: Pinworm infection is diagnosed by cellophane tape test collecting eggs around the perianal region in the morning. Enterobius causes perianal itching, especially in children. Eggs are oval, flattened on one side. Stool exams may miss eggs. Good hygiene and antihelminthic therapy prevent reinfection.

Q390. Answer: B

Explanation: S. haematobium resides in vesical veins, causing hematuria and bladder wall fibrosis. Eggs with terminal spines appear in urine. S. mansoni and S. japonicum affect intestines and liver. Transmission occurs through skin penetration by cercariae in contaminated water. Control includes snail eradication and improved sanitation.

Q391. Answer: B

Explanation: QC verifies analytical accuracy and precision by monitoring control materials with known values. It detects shifts, trends, or random errors before reporting results. QC is a core part of quality assurance programs. High test volumes or administrative efforts alone do not guarantee reliability or accuracy in patient testing.

Q392. Answer: C

Explanation: PT involves external agencies providing unknown specimens for analysis to assess a lab's accuracy compared to peer results. It ensures compliance with regulatory bodies like CLIA and CAP. Calibration adjusts instruments, validation tests new methods, and training focuses on personnel competency rather than performance benchmarking.

Q393. Answer: A

Explanation: Levey-Jennings charts plot control results versus time to identify random errors, shifts, or systematic trends in test performance. Data outside ±2 SD signals potential analytical problems requiring corrective action. These charts provide visual quality monitoring essential to maintain consistent laboratory accuracy and reliability.

Q394. Answer: A

Explanation: Westgard multirule system interprets Levey-Jennings chart data statistically (e.g., 1:2s, 2:2s, R:4s) to detect random or systematic analytical errors early. Violations trigger corrective actions before reporting results. It's fundamental in high-complexity testing. Reagent dating and staff documentation are unrelated to statistical QC interpretation.

Q395. Answer: A

Explanation: Scheduled preventive maintenance-cleaning, calibration checks, and part replacement-prevents unexpected instrument failure, ensuring consistent performance. Documentation supports accreditation compliance. It's proactive, reducing downtime and costly repairs. Regular servicing extends equipment lifespan and supports uninterrupted diagnostic operations critical for patient care.

Q396. Answer: D

Explanation: Chain of custody ensures specimen integrity in forensic, toxicology, and paternity testing by documenting every transfer from collection to reporting. Each handler signs and timestamps custody records. Routine medical testing doesn't require this strict tracking. Proper chain of custody safeguards admissibility of laboratory evidence in court.

Q397. Answer: A
Explanation: OSHA enforces workplace safety standards, including chemical hygiene, bloodborne pathogen protection, and hazard communication (MSDS/SDS use). Compliance ensures safe laboratory environments. HIPAA governs confidentiality, while accreditation falls under CLIA or CAP. OSHA training and documentation are mandatory for all laboratory employees handling biological or chemical hazards.
Q398. Answer: B
Explanation: BSCs use laminar airflow and HEPA filtration to protect personnel, specimen, and environment from infectious aerosols. Class II BSCs are standard for clinical microbiology. They must be certified annually. Proper technique and sash positioning maintain containment efficiency. BSCs are essential for biosafety levels 2 and above.
Q399. Answer: D
Explanation: Standard precautions assume all human specimens contain pathogens, requiring PPE (gloves, gowns, masks), safe sharps handling, and hand hygiene after each contact. This universal approach protects both personnel and patients. Selective PPE or conditional hygiene violates biosafety principles and increases infection risk.
Q400. Answer: A
Explanation: RCA systematically investigates incidents or errors to uncover fundamental process failures rather than assigning blame. It promotes corrective and preventive actions (CAPA) to prevent recurrence. Repeating tests or QC review doesn't address systemic issues. RCA is a core quality management tool in laboratory accreditation standards.

Made in the USA
Monee, IL
05 October 2026

64905541R00063